FIT FOR SEX

A Man's Guide to Enhancing and Maintaining Peak Sexual Performance

JOHN KNUTILA

REWARD BOOKS

Library of Congress Cataloging in Publication Data

Knutila, John.
    Fit for sex : a man's guide to peak sexual performance, potency,
and pleasure / John Knutila.
        p.   cm.
    ISBN 0-7352-0067-X (pbk.) — ISBN 0-13-975228-5
    1. Sex instruction for men. 2. Men—Sexual behavior. 3. Men—Health and hygiene.
I. Title.
HQ36.K58 1999
613.9'6'081—dc21   99-36948
                                                         CIP

© 2000 by Reward Books

Printed in the United States of America

10 9 8 7 6 5 4 3 2 1   10 9 8 7 6 5 4 3 2 1

ISBN 0-7352-0067-X (pbk.)   ISBN 0-13-975228-5

REWARD BOOKS
Paramus, NJ 07652

On the World Wide Web at http://www.phdirect.com

A NOTE TO THE READER:

This book is intended to inform men about many aspects of their sexual health and fitness. The ideas and suggestions included are not intended as a substitute for consulting with a doctor. All matters regarding health require proper diagnosis and treatment by a qualified health professional.

CONTENTS

INTRODUCTION

This book is a man's guide to creating and maintaining peak sexual fitness.

In the following pages, you'll find many ways to boost your sexual performance, pleasure, and health. An easy-to-use A-to-Z format presents clear tips and techniques for how to:

- Enjoy firm self-confidence in every erotic encounter.
- Introduce new arousal techniques to fan erotic fires.
- Give—and get—increasingly intense orgasms.
- Discover the #1 exercise to boost your sexual stamina.
- Soar beyond limiting attitudes and emotions.
- Use foods, herbs, and vitamins to nourish your sexuality.
- Enrich your overall health and well-being with the power of sex.

First let's answer the most obvious question: What is sexual fitness? One man's definition is five nightly orgasms. Another focuses on making his wife pregnant; yet a third, simply achieving an erection. Ultimately, each man has his own definition, which will change over the course of his lifetime.

So sexual fitness can mean agility, potency, endurance, grooming, confidence—the list quickly moves beyond the physical. And not surprisingly. Because any man with his head on straight knows that sex happens between people, not just bodies. Emotions and attitudes loom large in today's sexuality. **This book defines sexual fitness as a man's body, mind, and emotions healthy and fully engaged in each sexual encounter.** The result is optimum performance, satisfying intimacy, and unfailing confidence.

Experience the heights of sexual fitness now—being in the flow, in the fun, and in the pleasure of being fully male and fully alive.

We're talking peak performance and satisfaction here—planting-your-feet-on-the-carpet, hooting, rip-snorting radical well-being. And the full spectrum of more subtle versions on the sunny side of sex.

What you won't find here is moralizing about what to do, when, or with whom. Read on and explore the endless potential for optimum sex in your life today. And tomorrow. There's a lot of ground to cover, so let's get started.

Gentlemen, start your engines.

AFTERPLAY

Life is good.

Head on pillow, you're staring at the ceiling, smiling and puffing lazily on a cigarette. "That was incredible," she murmurs.

OK, forget the cigarette if you don't smoke (and needless to say, you shouldn't). But you know the feeling. It's called *afterglow*. But don't get lost in your own satisfaction, Buster. There are many good reasons why that picture, if it's not too clouded with smoke or ego, should also include *afterplay*. Why? To answer that, let's digress momentarily into the science of sex. This won't take long, so stick with it. You'll be glad you did.

A MOUNTAIN OF SEX

Many sex experts divide lovemaking into four stages: excitement, plateau, orgasm, and resolution.

Consider sex as a hike up a mountain. The ascent is called excitement, the broad mountain top is a plateau, with a peak or peaks called orgasm, and coming down the other side is resolution.

The important point to remember is this: males and females experience sexual hikes differently. Women generally need more time on the way up, are more likely to find several peaks, and need longer coming down. It's the descent—afterplay—that we're exploring now.

The fact is, women remain physically and emotionally involved with sex longer than men. You might be finished and done, ready for a can of beer or the late movie, but she's still wandering down the mountain, enjoying the view and the smell of wildflowers—and expecting your company along the way. It takes longer for her heart rate, her circulation, and muscles to return to normal. Remember, good sex is reciprocal. From that viewpoint, respecting her needs is good form. Good for her, and good for you.

MINING EMOTIONAL GOLD

This book is about being sexually fit in every way. The hallmark of afterplay is emotion. Physically, you're spent. Mentally, you're who knows where? But emotionally, there's much to be said for being connected with your partner.

1

Of course that's not a hard and fast rule. But once you understand her needs, and she realizes you do too, good things are on the way. Remember, the next time you're looking to wander up the mountain, whether in ten minutes or ten days, her reaction might be based on her last descent.

Keep in touch—literally. You've just visited the magic place called sex. Your job now is to enhance her return journey. What do you get out of it? The expansiveness—the expanded pleasure—of the moment. Also, look into that dimly lit area within called emotions. If you'd like more of the one called confidence, now's a great time to create it. Drink deeply from the tap of afterplay. If you have questions about sex, the open atmosphere of afterplay makes them appropriate. Of course, openness means vulnerability, so this is not the time for criticism. But as you humbly acknowledge the pleasure and performance just passed, you bolster confidence. It's only natural.

WHEN AFTERSHOCK REPLACES AFTERPLAY

Let's face it, sex isn't always great. In fact, sometimes it stinks. Maybe you just couldn't get those office politics off your mind. Or maybe one or both of you is tired and just going through the motions. So it wasn't memorable. Now what?

Every act of love can't be textbook perfect. Leave room for spontaneity. Cut yourself some slack. Crack a joke. Communicate. Saying a little is a lot better than saying nothing.

Don't feel guilty if you feel like sleeping. Often for some of us—and occasionally for most—sleep is the natural final chapter to sex. The tension's off. The exertion's over. Fine. But unless you sink into dreamland immediately after orgasm, just a few loving words or caresses go a long way. She needs to be understanding too. Just don't get into the habit of turning your back on her and dialing out for pizza immediately after the action subsides.

Conversely, there's the aftershock, the shocked silence, following your inability to "perform." What follows that says a lot about the relationship, which, in one important sense, is defined by how a couple reacts when things aren't picture perfect. Many women don't understand a man's needs in this moment. Consider yourself lucky if the one you're with does. Either way, communication is the answer. Begin with what you're feeling. Don't start blaming her. And don't blame yourself either. Blame is a one way ticket to nowhere. Sharing your feelings is a great way to build intimacy, and intimacy is the royal road to great sex and enhanced satisfaction. So after-shock can definitely be a cloud with a silver lining.

EIGHT TIPS FOR GREAT AFTERPLAY

Tune In, Don't Drop Out

Unless you're super tired and slip into dreamland immediately after orgasm, there's no excuse for rolling off a woman and into your own private world. As this chapter has stressed, afterplay is a special time, a perfect opportunity to build intimacy and confidence. If it feels like a chore, you might want to reconsider why you're having sex with this partner, or why you're having sex at all. Maybe masturbation is more appropriate to your immediate needs. If not, enjoy some or all of the following.

Touch and Feel

Two methods of sharing are supremely appropriate: talk and touch. Each has its place and time. Sometimes nothing needs to be said. Touching or caressing say it all. Great. Other times a gentle compliment or comment or question are right. Also great. Explore her needs and express yours. Just remember that you're both naked in more ways than one. Enjoy the after-glow. Save the searchlight of criticism for some other time.

Kiss

Kissing is as natural here as any other part of sex. How better to express appreciation, connection, satisfaction, or for that matter, love? And who knows what kissing will lead to?

Eat

Hey, you're hungry. No problem. Eating is good. The key is not forgetting her. Now is a great time to keep your connection strong, whether in bed or in the kitchen. Maybe you can go the extra mile and forego wolfing down the hoagie and beer in the kitchen, and instead bring some food and drink back to bed for her. There aren't any rules, thank God. It's just about connection and intimacy in whatever form they take.

Joke

Humor can be a great release of tension, a bridge, an inroad to areas not otherwise easily broached. Use it! Respond to it! Even if you've just felt mountains move, humor can be a natural reaction. Just be sure you're laughing with her, not at her.

Turn on the TV

Speaking of mountains moving, afterplay, like sex in general, doesn't always have to be monumental. The connection can be continued in little ways as well, like watching a television program or a video. Stay close. Stay entwined. Or gently transition from sex back to life in general.

Bathe Together

What a classic! A bath or a shower hold excellent, sudsy potential for togetherness. It's a great way to get to know each other, for the first time or as if for the first time. Whether it's massage-like or simply a wash on the way to the kitchen, like everything else regarding afterplay, it's less *what* you do than *how*.

Rub-a-dub-dub, two lovers in the tub!

Foreplay

We've come full circle. Having discussed some more mundane forms of afterplay, now here's the magic—when the sheer ardor and excitement overflows one act of love and spills into the next. The thrusting, moaning spasms have subsided, only to build again after a pause. Afterplay here is merely a resting place in the journey, inseparable from foreplay and intercourse. It's all lovemaking. A different pace and intensity outwardly, perhaps, but inwardly connected by mutual attraction and the desire it provokes. When the love is strong, the distinction between afterplay and the rest of life becomes small. Now you're talking big intimacy. Big satisfaction. And big love.

APHRODISIACS

How do deer testicles relate to pine nuts and black panties?

You guessed it—they're aphrodisiacs. Or at least they're *reputed* to be aphrodisiacs. And there's the rub. Exactly what's fact and fiction here? We need to know because we're talking torrid turn-ons and eye-popping feats of sexual athletics here. Or so one would think after hearing numerous reports from the wonderful world of aphrodisiacs.

Let's keep our feet on the ground and start with a definition. Broadly speaking, an aphrodisiac is anything that arouses or intensifies sexual desire or sexual response. Hundreds of herbs, drugs, foods, and objects qualify. In this book, drugs prescribed for impotence are discussed in the *Erectile Dysfunction* chapter, so look there for news about the much-discussed Viagra.

So which aphrodisiacs work? And more to the point, *which will work for you this weekend*?

Depends on who you ask. The FDA throws cold water on the whole subject by endorsing no aphrodisiac, even though they do sanction drugs for erectile dysfunction. But of course they want cold facts derived from precise studies in sterile laboratories.

On the other hand, friendly marketers urge you to try their "miraculous" products like pheromone perfumes and herbal supplements. Their products definitely get results—to the tune of hundreds of millions in sales. More on their ingredients below.

And then there's the folklore—shiploads of exotic tales about erotic magic achieved with this potion or that plant.

Who's a guy to believe?

> ### Side Effects? Yes please!
>
> According to the Canadian Journal of Psychiatry (November 1993), some users of the antidepressant drug Clomipramine have reported an interesting side effect: patients of both sexes have experienced spontaneous orgasms as the result of *yawning*. Unfortunately, most people taking the drug report only reduced libido. But roughly 5% of its users have presumably shelved their coffee cups and found new enthusiasm for those early morning staff meetings.

PICK YOUR PLEASURE

Casanova loved his oysters. The French use onion soup. Finding *your* ideal aphrodisiac depends on your sexual preferences, your condition, your expectations, and obviously, good ol' experimentation. Hey, it's tough work, but someone—in this case you—has to do it. Step one is defining what you're after.

First, whose response are you trying to boost? Consider the desire factor. If a sexual relationship is hampered by one partner having a substantially lower sex drive than the other, it could be reasonable for the partner with less desire to try an aphrodisiac while the other doesn't.

But in today's world, a man focused on bolstering his own pleasure with no concern for his partner's will do fine—if he's in the arms of a prostitute. Otherwise he's living in the past or a fantasy world. Even before considering the pure selfishness of it, we know he's missing a very important point: when arousal is the goal, a partner filled with beckoning, radiant desire is a super-premium aphrodisiac.

So building her desire along with yours is paramount. Some standbys for that purpose, like chocolate, are classics for getting her focused on the matter at hand. Alternatively, champagne has long been associated with putting both partners in the mood for love.

With such a vast array of sex-enhancing candidates to choose from, let's first get a handle on how they're grouped.

FIVE FAMILIES OF APHRODISIACS

This section includes classic as well as up-and-coming aphrodisiacs. By understanding how each works you'll know how to categorize all those not listed here. And you should get a sense of which to consider and which to avoid and why. Each has its own lesson.

The Legends of Pre-History

If you're looking for an aphrodisiac, join the club: males the world over have had the same impulse for thousands of years. Early versions sound suspiciously simple, and highlight an important point. By eating seal penises, tiger testicles, or plants resembling the human versions, one taps the power of *association and assimilation*: what you eat is what you get. So why not simply ingest whatever makes bulls powerful, for instance, or rabbits prolific?

Aphrodisiacs Short List:

- The Legends of Pre-History
- Herbs and Spices
- Pharmaceuticals
- Food
- Miscellaneous

And who knows, maybe they worked (and judging by contemporary trade in endangered species, still work) in some way modern science can't fathom. Three contemporary examples are ginseng; with its human-like root; rhinoceros horn, with its super-phallic shape; and oysters, which glorifies

> **Strong-Like-Bull Department**
> Why search the animal kingdom for what you already have? One source estimates that 500 pounds of bull testicle extract equals an average dose of human male sex hormones.[1]

feminine delights to come while delivering a mega dose of zinc.[2]

Power can be created by belief itself. Traditions enliven the power of positive thinking. If you believe a rhino horn holds power, that belief may create power. This is confirmed by modern studies of aphrodisiacs and the power of placebos. But who can justify the slaughter of any animal, let alone an endangered one, for a sex-enhancer, when so many options are available today?

Herbs and Spices

There are a number of herbs with amorous reputations. Hundreds of commercial preparations and mixtures are available. Satisfied users report impressive results, while critics of the industry cry fraud. Once again, the only way to find out which, if any, work for you is to experiment. Enthusiasts recommend combining and varying aphrodisiacs, so as not to wear out the effects of any one. Some have side effects in various forms, so consult with your doctor or qualified herbal health professional to make sure you stay on the safe side of aphrodisiacs such as:

Yohimbe Derived from the bark of an African tree called yohimbe (and quebracho, a South American tree), this herb has a long history for use in ceremonies requiring sexual stamina. Its active ingredient—yohimbine—is available in prescription form for treating erectile dysfunction. It has the distinction of being the only herb so approved by the FDA. But the FDA disputes claims that yohimbine boosts sexual desire.

Yohimbine's alkaloids stimulate nerves, increase neurotransmitters, and have a vasodilating effect on the circulatory system, which allows enhanced blood flow to the genitals, in this case producing firm erections, but heightened sensations for women as well. It is available in nonprescription herbal form in health food stores. But even herbal authority James Duke recommends the prescription form over the herbal to avoid side effects.[3]

Ginseng   Ginseng has a long history of use in Asia as a popular general tonic. It also has a reputation as an aphrodisiac. Like Yohimbine, it's associated with increasing blood flow to the penis, though by different chemical means. Ginseng is thought to enhance the amount of nitric oxide, which has a vasodilating effect in the penis. Among the safest aphrodisiacs, its effects require weeks or months of use to take effect.

Ginkgo Biloba   Extracted from the leaves of a large deciduous tree that is one of the oldest existing trees on earth, Ginkgo has been shown to help people suffering from Alzheimer's disease. It does so by increasing blood flow to the brain, and can do the same for the penis. One study showed ginkgo restoring erections to 50% of the participants.[4] As with Ginseng, however, the effects are not immediate, but can take months to realize.

Spices   Like coffee, which has been cited for its stimulating, and aphrodisiac effect, several spices have been claimed to boost amorous feelings, such as cloves, ginger, anise, cardamom, cinnamon, nutmeg, and saffron. They of course figure heavily into the fourth category of aphrodisiacs below, food and its preparation.

Pharmaceuticals and Supplements

A vast variety of pharmaceutical drugs can impair sexual functioning; antidepressants and antihypertensives are foremost among them. But more and more drugs are finding new life as sex-enhancing medications.

Spanish Fly

Everyone's heard variations of the legend: The boyfriend slips some Spanish Fly into his girlfriend's soda. She satisfies him on lover's lane, then proceeds to satisfy herself on the gearshift knob, the seatback, his elbow, etc. for long hours afterwards.

In reality the legend has a dark side. The active ingredient in Spanish Fly is cantharidin, a chemical found in a beetle from southern Europe, and which in small concentrations can blister skin. Far from being a magical love potion, it can be toxic. By irritating the gastrointestinal and urinary tract, it produces erections and a pseudo sexual drive. Adverse reactions range from nausea, priapism, seizures, and possibly death, making this is a good substance to avoid.

Viagra was originally tested to treat heart-disease chest pain. When the drug was almost rejected, a doctor noticed reports of a now well-known, prominent side effect, and millions of formerly impotent men have smiles on their faces as a result. Other pharmaceutical drugs have produced similar surprises.

Two prominent examples are the Alzheimer's drug deprenyl and anti-Parkinson's drugs containing L-dopa. Their intriguing side effects include increased sexual desire.

Non-prescription supplements also have their fans. Niacin, or B-3, has a growing reputation as a sex enhancer. It produces a flush on the skin which can magnify the erotic sensations naturally occurring for both men and women.

And an amino acid called L-argentine is said to increase the nitric oxide in blood, which has positive results for erections. It can also increase desire and arousal in women.

Food

Curious cavemen, ancient Greeks, and today's man on the street all have considered various foods to be sex boosters. Again, the evidence is anecdotal, not scientific. But some things are beyond the realm of science. Like that indescribable sense of well-being after a meal that magically translates into passion as a romantic evening wears on.

Take oysters. Beyond their erotic texture, what's up with their powerful aphrodisiac reputation? Is it the zinc content, or their low-fat, high-protein composition? Whatever the chemistry, they work for some, and that's what counts. And who's to argue with the sexual prowess of oyster-loving Casanova? Walnuts, onions, pine nuts, apricots, chocolate—many foods have strong reputations as aphrodisiacs.

But perhaps as important as specific biochemicals in particular foods is how they all work together when carefully prepared and presented in the sensual collection of smells, aromas, tastes, and textures called a meal. Cooking and eating, especially when lovingly shared, have the power to return us to the present—and into the presence of our lovers. Gone are our workaday pressures and worries. In their place are the culinary delights where our own awareness slowly transforms mere vegetables, spices, fruits, and more into the sensuous and erotic.

APHRODISIACS IN THE WORLD

By the time 5:00 Friday rolled around, Jim was more than ready to set sail from the office. In fact, he had high hopes for a special night with his girl-friend Gina, who had invited him to her house for dinner for what she called an aphrodisiac evening. On the way he stopped at the wine store and the video rental shop.

She greeted him at the door with a long kiss and an intriguing scent which had him changing gears before he crossed her threshold. He asked about it and Gina said it was sandalwood. He noticed on the way into her kitchen she had a candle-lit table set in her dining room.

The best aphrodisiac money can't buy

Exercise may be the cheapest and most reliable aphrodisiac of all. As we'll see later in the book, exercise and cardiovascular health are close-ly related, and firm erections are strongly connected with healthy blood flow. Also, exercise can increase pain-relieving, feel-good brain chemicals called endorphins, making us more receptive to erotic impulses from within and without.

She got a plate of oysters ready while he opened the bottle of champagne he had brought and poured two flutes. They settled by a fire in the living room and by the time the champagne and oysters were gone, they were nibbling on each other's ears as well. Jim felt his desire flowing and by the way she was kissing he knew she did too.

They went back into the kitchen and talked while she pulled together a show-stopping meal of lobster and truffles, followed by fresh peaches and apricots with chocolate shaved over them. As they ate, the food and flickering candlelight and her full lips and rosy skin had Jim sitting on the edge of his seat and feeling like he was floating slightly above it and toward Gina. After the meal they settled in the living room for a movie. He produced the video a clerk had recommended when he inquired about an erotic film. It was made by a woman and actually had a plot, along with some extremely arous-ing sex scenes. They both began exploring each other with their hands and lips, and didn't make it through the movie before undressing. She had on creme-colored lace underwear that made him feel like exploding. They started slow and spent an hour making passionate love on pillows and throws thrown on the carpet. Afterward they laughed when Jim mentioned a small bottle of herbal aphrodisiac he had brought along.

"Maybe next week," Gina cooed as she fell asleep in his arms in front of him as they lay naked like spoons in front of the fire.

ATTITUDES

"Sexual fitness—that's about the body, right?" Well, yes, a healthy and well-conditioned body contributes to great sex. But mental attitudes figure in too—big time. After all, more and more experts refer to the brain as the largest male sex organ.

Strange thought? Not at all; the mind is where arousal often begins. A memory, a fantasy, or an arousing sight, sound, or smell send a call to action from the brain through the nervous system to the other sex organs. Direct contact with the penis (as in touching, holding, rubbing) reverses that process, but even there, sex is a balance between cues coming in and thoughts and emotions directing response from the inside.

Sexual fitness is inseparable from mental fitness. And mental fitness is conditioned by mental attitudes, those fixed ideas we all carry around that determine how we approach any given situation. Regarding sex, we all come out of childhood with a mix of attitudes, some positive, some not.

Question: who among us had an upbringing free of distortion about sex; had all his questions answered honestly and correctly, never felt ashamed or guilty about sex in any way, and had only caring, enlightened sexual partners? Answer: no one.

The good news is that sexual attitudes are flexible, and changeable. We all have something to learn—and unlearn—about sex. Accepting both leads to less stress, better relationships, and better overall health. And better sex too.

MOVE ONWARD MENTALLY—TO GREAT SEX

Maybe you wish your penis was bigger. Or harder. You wish your lover was more passionate, or you were getting it more often, or sex could be as exciting now as it once was.

What if. Why not. If only. The old sexual wish list. Where does it come from anyway? The answer is simple: the past. From your parents, your junior high school locker room, skin mags, or the TV screen. When you think about it, many of our attitudes are pretty stale, one-dimensional, laughable even. And in need of a tuneup.

It's important to recognize and accept your attitudes about sex, whatever they are. That's the first step. If some of them need change, that's the second step.

Becoming conscious of our own attitudes is easy if we're in a love relationship. Negative attitudes surface there sooner or later, causing suffering and unhappiness, either in you or your partner. There's no better indication of an attitude in need of review than mental discomfort.

It's not easy to change an attitude. We all resist change. That's natural. But when there's an important relationship on the line, not to mention sex, the incentive is strong.

THE MENTAL FOUNDATION FOR GOOD SEX

No, it's not a tax shelter in Nevada. The mental foundation for good sex is four attitudes on which healthy sexual relationships are built. Of course every man has his own definition of good sex. This book proposes that sexual fitness today is dedicated to the proposition that:

Sexual Partners are Equal

In most circles, Macho Man has gone the way of Neanderthal Man. And good riddance. But don't mistake sexual equality with reduced masculinity. It takes more of a man to regard a woman as his equal than not. In the wonderful dance of healthy sex, no matter who's leading, male and female are equal. Way different, but equal.

Good Sex is Consensual

Mutual consent between adults is the very basis of healthy sexual relations, even the kinky kind. Those who disagree need help. Period. This should be too obvious to mention, but unfortunately abuse and rape statistics show otherwise.

Good Sex is Healthy

This isn't a moral statement. Sexual fitness is not only part of overall health, it helps create and maintain it. Respecting your sexuality and that of others is a requirement for full sexual fitness.

Good Sex is About Pleasure, Not Performance

Expectations, real or imagined, can push or pull us to approach sex unrealistically. For a man, acknowledging that he is not a sex machine but a human being, complete with strengths and limitations, thoughts and emotions, is not easy. But accepting it will lead to highter levels of well-being, sexual and otherwise. As we discuss elsewhere in this book, focusing on intercourse at the expense of arousal is a common and troublesome attitude which many men need to unlearn in working through sexual problems.

SEVEN ATTITUDES THAT FAN THE SENSUAL FIRES

Built on that foundation are seven other mental attitudes that can transform going-through-the-motions into sexual delight and fulfillment.

Be Curious

It may have killed the cat, but curiosity enlivens a man and his sexuality. Without it, an erotic relationship flies on autopilot. How can we discover a woman's desires, or remain aware of how they change, without being curious?

The rewards of curiosity are many. In a relationship, it shows you care, and nothing means more to a woman emotionally than that. Curiosity nourishes your connection, emotionally and physically. And it's not something you need to invent. The trick is simply to remain responsive to your innate curiosity. Take the quiz below to gauge whether you're letting routines or inner constraints hold you back.

Be Tolerant

Tolerating differences in other people is a sign of strength. When you're sexually tolerant, your lover can be herself. That's a powerful gift, but one that's not always easy to give.

Test Your CQ (Curiosity Quotient)

- Do you know the last book your lover read?
- When was the last time you asked your lover about oral sex, or about how you could improve your technique?
- If your lover flew to a city two thousand miles away, to what store would she first go?
- What is your lover's main sexual worry?
- If your lover could change one thing about you, what would it be?

If you don't know the answer to any (or, heaven forbid, all) of these questions, why not ask?

Tolerance takes emotional strength, which, like muscular strength, can be developed. Listen to feedback. Entertain criticism seriously. Keep an open mind and believe in yourself.

Is she asking you to talk more than you want? Well, give it a try. See what it's like. Try describing why you don't feel the need to talk all the time. Maybe you can do it, maybe you can't. It's the effort that counts most. Hey, often in life we profit the most from things we wouldn't have chosen if left to ourselves. And there lies the greatest gift of tolerance: by giving something up, if only an attitude, we get something back in return. And just possibly something better.

Try Optimism

Some men just seem to gravitate to the dark view. They figure they'll choose the door hiding a tiger, or will pick the stock bound to plunge. Why not try a walk on the sunny side? Use the power of visualization. Picture what you want (not what you fear) and maybe you'll get it! Optimists tend toward the relaxed approach; pessimists tend to tense up. Women pick up on a positive attitude. Their radar senses it. So be positive. It'll give you a leg up.

Cultivate Presence

You'll be less stressed and more relaxed. You'll be more connected emotionally. You'll be more open to sensations. Many good things pull you into the present: prayer, meditation, exercise, and massage, to name a few. You'll find others throughout this book.

Be Creative

That means be willing to risk. Explore. And occasionally fail. Touch her with your tongue. Make love on a chair. Transform your kisses into sucking. Blow air. Nibble. It's active curiosity. Become a creative legend in your own bed.

Trust Humor

Sex doesn't need to be heavy. Hey, why not chuckle your way into ecstasy? Humor can be a great inlet to serious action and serious involvement. But don't hide behind it. Nothing is more boring than a man who armors himself with constant, sex-saturated ditties and puns. Reveal something about yourself. Lose the poker face. Have some fun!

Value Intimacy

Intimacy underlies deeply satisfying sex. Sure, every erotic encounter can't be a grand opera of rapturous moans and intricate positions. Hey, a quickie always has its place. But without a background of respect, closeness, and trust, sex remains a matter of friction and tension reduction. Sure, we're drawn to a woman's body and the lacy things that glorify it. And we get hot and bothered just thinking about the sexual possibilities they promise. But we're separated from deeper satisfaction when unable to move beyond the superficial. Yes, there's a place for all levels of connection. But to really ring her bell and yours, go with the naked truth of intimacy.

Long-term Attitudes for Losers

Me first.
Soap! Who needs it?
I'm right. You're wrong.
Sorry, I don't wash dishes.
You'll do like I tell you.
Leave me alone.
Let's do it.

Long-term Attitudes for Winners

I'm listening.
Can I help?
Who are you in there?
Here's what I'm feeling.
Tell me what you like.
Let's take our time here.
Let's make love

COMMUNICATION

"You know how to whistle, don't you Steve?"

Bogart is tinkering with his fishing reel, trying to concentrate on doing the right thing. But there's Lauren Bacall in a robe, slender and dark-eyed at his hotel room door. She purrs an answer to her own question: "You just put your lips together and blow." With that, Bogie's ties to the independent life are deep-sixed. The year was 1944 and the film is *To Have and Have Not*. Any man who doubts the power of erotic communication should check it out.

CONVEY YOUR NEEDS

Communication. A stuffy word with a dry definition: "to convey information." But it sure adds spice to sex. Just think of all the ways *sexual* information gets conveyed. A look, a loaded comment, a kiss, or the whole nine yards. Let's start with the verbal kind and then explore the rest.

Obviously, Lauren Bacall's point isn't instructions for whistling. She's conveying interest, availability, and desire. Seduction—sexual enticement—derives its power from indirectness. That can be powerful, and powerfully enjoyable. More on that in the *Seduction* section.

It's the other, direct kind of sharing that has earned males the reputation of being communication non-events. Sharing sexual needs and preferences is the real-life stuff beyond cinematic happy endings. Is *your* communication style helping you along the path to great sex?

Sex therapists say that a good sexual relationship usually includes good communication. That makes sense. From the get-go, you're here and she's there, and once you're past the frenzied-mutual-strip phase, you'll need a two-way bridge to share emotions, needs, and preferences. Take communication seriously and you're on the road to sexual gold. Ignore it and you're likely to feel a nagging discontent, from within—and from the woman in your life. Sure, you could go out and find a new one, but guess what, you'll more than likely find yourself in the same boat regarding her need to talk. So be careful before making any moves based on her pestering you about what you're feeling—unless you're headed for a monastery and a vow of silence.

MASTER THE COMMUNICATION GAME

In his book *Between People: Communicating One-to-One*, John Stanford likens communication between the sexes to a game of catch. Picture this: you and your lover are on the beach. You throw her a ball (let's make it a classic beach ball). She catches it and throws it back. Simple, right? Now substitute thoughts and/or feelings for the ball and, well, you get the idea.

If both parties aren't involved, communication evaporates. But when the game is on, you listen to what she's saying, entertain it, and respond. She does the same, the process continues, and pretty soon you're both enjoying the fruits of understanding. Satisfying connections follow—of minds, emotions, and bodies.

Since it sounds simple in theory, why is it so hard in reality? Sometimes it's just a matter of being lost in *assumptions*. "She should know what I want," "I should know what she wants," etc. Whoa! Now you're in the shadowy realm of *Should*, a place of little light and much frustration.

Ask! Tell! Give the ball a gentle toss. And by all means if she does so, catch it and toss it back. Remember, communication is a skill and can be learned like any other. It takes practice to listen well. Pretty soon you'll trade the beach ball for a football and handle deep passes with ease.

Defensiveness is another hurdle. "What do you mean it tickles when I kiss your neck? That's not *my* fault!" Maybe her neck is just plain ticklish. Again, ask. If you care about each other, sincere communication will only help, no matter how uncomfortable at first. And if you don't care about each other, you might inquire why you're together in the first place.

Cut yourself some slack. No one said communication is easy, but the rewards are great. The process goes on indefinitely. Even if you're with the same woman for years, you'll both change physically, mentally, and emotionally, and keeping up with the changes requires communication.

SIX TIPS FOR EFFECTIVE TALKING —AND LISTENING

Talk About Sex When Not in Bed

Generally it's a good idea to keep sack-time free from involved discussions about sex. Communicate with your touch and ardor, unless you're with an intellectual who is turned on by analysis. In that case, bring a volume of Kierkegaard to bed!

Acknowledge and Reward Communication Breakthroughs

This goes for both of you as you push into uncharted territory of sharing. Positive feedback creates motivation to continue, and excel. And it sure feels good.

Share Feelings About the Simplest of Sexual Topics First

You'd be surprised how grateful a woman can be for your openness. By starting simple, you avoid defensiveness and create success. Concentrate on what *you* want or need or feel, and encourage her to reciprocate.

Stick to Specifics

Don't dwell in generalities when discussing fine points. When you're specific about something, you're conveying useful information. The more indirect you are, the more you encourage misinterpretation. "Your teeth hurt my penis," is much more useful than "Be more careful."

Set Aside a Few Minutes for Intimate Monologue

A goofy contradiction in terms? No. When one of you talks and the other listens, it's great practice in active listening, and a great way to get the heavier stuff off your chest. Don't be put off by the difficulty in starting; it might take a few minutes to get to the heart of the matter. Don't bore her with chatter, or offend her with criticism. Be honest.

See a Professional Counselor if Needed

This is a good idea, plain and simple. Lessons speed advances in skiing and multimedia—why not communication? A good counselor is an objective party, and is trained to see where you're holding back and why. If you haven't experienced it, you'd be amazed how great the process feels.

COMMUNICATION SUPERCHARGERS

Sometimes we think we're communicating wonderfully when we're really not.[5] Here are a few suggestions for improving your style of sharing in and out of the sack.

Let Her Finish Her Sentences

You're not really listening when you interrupt her in mid-sentence. You might think your thought is too important to delay, but that might just be your take. How to know? Ask her. Maybe your comment was justified. or maybe it wasn't. She'll tell you one way or the other. Listen when she does.

Don't Laugh Your Way Through a Serious Topic

Sure, it may seem funny to you, but that doesn't mean it is to her. And if it isn't, you've thrown a wrench in the gears. Of course humor is delightful in its place, but don't use it as a hiding place.

Don't Assume She Knows What You Feel or Think

Whether in the office or the bedroom, one of the easiest communication mistakes is to assume that someone else knows what you know, or has even understood what you just said. Take the time to express your needs. And take the time to listen to hers. And by all means don't blame her if she doesn't know something you assume she does.

Say What You Mean and Mean What You Say

Of course there's a time for indirectness and innuendo. But not every time you open your mouth. And not when something important needs to be shared. Remember, this is not easy stuff. You might have to seek help in learning how to communicate, because you might have deep reasons for not being able to communicate effectively. Okay, then it's time to explore them, with a therapist if necessary. No blame. But with so much to gain, why not make the effort? If you really care about her, and she cares about you, communication is critical, and hopefully, enjoyable too. Talk with someone who can help, or ask a bookseller to point you in the direction of a good book on the subject, such as John Gray's *Men are From Mars, Women Are From Venus* series.

HOW TO MOVE BEYOND WORDS

In sex, as elsewhere, there's a point when words only go so far. There's a limit to what can or should be said verbally, and there's good reason for turning to touch. That reason is intimacy.

Many studies highlight the importance of intimacy for our well-being from infancy onward. Unless you're a tall, thin, cigar-chewing cowboy in a spaghetti western, you have a need for intimacy. Being able to recognize and value it is a major prerequisite for full sexual fitness.

Conversely, you might choose to hide in aloof macho detachment. But like water finding a way downhill, the need for intimacy will find a way into your consciousness, despite attempts to deny it with behavior better suited to war than love and sex. When we decide instead on the road to intimacy, sexual signals and touch are important parts of the trip.

SIX HIGH-PRIORITY SEXUAL SIGNALS

Sending and receiving sexual signals are early relationship high points. They rate high in terms of sheer exhilaration, and start the transformation from stranger to lover.

Sexual fitness includes comfort with both sending and receiving a range of sexual signals. The six that follow are phrased in terms of sending, but apply equally receiving:

Enter Her Territory

We all lay claim to a portion of the space around us. And we're very much aware when someone else enters it. So signal interest by entering her territory in a non-threatening way. On a deep level of her being, she'll know when and why you're there, and what your intentions are.

Make Eye Contact

Whether from near or far, making and holding eye contact is a very strong signal. Staring might not be polite, but it's potent. It's interesting how a non-verbal signal like this can say so much, so powerfully.

Smile

It's the universal good-will sign. A simple smile, alone or combined with any of these other signals, can be a beacon of intention. But don't paste a false smile on your face if there's no corresponding emotion within. These signals are about communication, not manipulation. Sooner or later, dishonest communication backfires.

Use Open Body Signals

Most everyone recognizes that crossed arms and legs aren't a signal of openness. So stand or sit in a more welcoming posture. But here, as elsewhere, there are exceptions. A "closed" posture might be more natural for you at first. So combining it with open eye contact might be perceived as natural, and honest—even funny. Experiment. Relax. Enjoy.

Use Conversational Touching

Putting a hand on her shoulder or forearm while talking might be the first physical contact you make. As such, the simple gesture gains import. And if welcomed, it easily leads to further stages of intimate touch.

Hold Hands

Remember the first time you held your first girlfriend's hand? Or put your arm around her in a movie theater? These gestures haven't lost any of their magic or their everyday power.

WHEN TO LET YOUR FINGERS DO THE TALKING

Peak lovemaking is more than a roll in the hay (although it can certainly include one). We need to tune into a woman's desires, understand them, and with time and attention, fan them into erotic fires. Touching, whether in or out of bed, is a powerful step in that process.

Initially, touching signals interest. Then it compliments the words which directly or indirectly signal desire. Finally it goes beyond words and takes communication to new heights in the intimate touching called sex.

Each stage has an appropriate touch. Hugging, massaging, caressing, kissing, stroking, and squeezing all have their own place—where the physical and emotional meet. Words are best for jealousy or anger. The emotions best expressed by sexual touch are affection and love. When you're ready to make love, switch to touch, and don't stop touching even when you've arrived at deep, mutual satisfaction.

COMMUNICATION IN THE WORLD

Bruce is a successful financial advisor. He and his wife Elaine, a teacher, have two young children. Professional and family demands have gradually reduced the amount of intimate time they spend together.

One night in bed, at the end of a typically long day, and after being rebuffed again by Elaine, Bruce angrily blurted out his frustration with too little sex. He threw off the covers, stomped out of the bedroom and spent the night on the living room sofa. Elaine didn't speak to him for three days, and refused to let him touch her for a week. Then she called a marriage counselor and made an appointment.

They knew they needed more open dialogue in their day-to-day lives, but one suggestion by their counselor surprised them: intimate monologue. Now, one night a week after the children are asleep, they each make a point to talk, uninterrupted, for fifteen minutes. It seemed hard at first, but became easier. For Bruce, it's a chance to express his frustrations with work, which he realizes have begun to motivate his wanting sex with Elaine whether or not she's interested. Elaine listens with interest. When she speaks, Bruce realizes by his strong urge to interrupt how his listening skills have weakened. This new communication has forged renewed intimacy, which has added renewed heat to their sex lives.

CONTRACEPTION

Suggestion: if you're trying to have children, turn to the fertility chapter. All others read on.

Good contraception is required in the modern world; required in our country not by law, but by the main idea fueling this book—total sexual fitness means being fit and prepared to fully engage in each sexual experience with mind, body, and emotions all present and accounted for.

Be prepared. Understand the methods and make an informed decision about which to use. Take responsibility. Men take responsibility, boys don't, and boys should stay with masturbation.

First, learn the options. We'll focus on those in which men take an active role.

The second step is planning ahead. Despite what some people say, contraceptives and passion are not mutually exclusive. And mature passion isn't burdened with anxiety about sexually transmitted diseases and unwanted pregnancies. Also, a woman is turned on by signs of caring, and being knowledgeable and prepared in this area is a definite sign that you care.

The third step is to use your method of choice consistently. Find the method that works best for you and your lover. All have pros and cons, and vary in how well they work. Effectiveness for each contraceptive method is measured in expected pregnancies in 100 women using it for one year. So during one year, if 1 woman out of 100 became pregnant using the pill, 99 would not. In that case, the pill would be rated 99% effective.

The range of contraceptive practices for men varies widely. We'll look at condoms, the rhythm method, coitus interruptus, and vasectomy. Whichever method you as man and partner decide on, commit yourself to it. Use it without fail. Let contraceptives help you explore the world of sex safely, responsibly—and passionately.

Condom

Use one with confidence—if you use it properly.

Mr. Sperm, wriggling through his microscopic world, measures only .003 mm in diameter, and STD organisms are smaller yet. The good news is that neither can fit through an intact latex condom.[6]

In controlled studies, condoms rate 98% effective or better. In the real world, however, failure rates average 12%. Why? Improper use, not using one every time, or failure of the condom itself. Let's look more closely at each.

There's more to using a condom properly than just putting it on before you ejaculate. First, put it on as soon as you're erect, and before intercourse, because your penis can release sperm before you ejaculate. For the same reason, before unrolling a condom, make sure you've got the proper side out the first time. Test with your fingers to make sure the inside of the rolled condom is against the head of your penis—you don't want to turn it around leaving even one sperm on the outside. It only unrolls one way so it's easy to tell. Uncircumcised males should pull back their foreskin before putting on a condom.

GETTING IT ON (AND OFF)

When rolling a condom on, squeeze the end, leaving a half-inch of loose space up front so the semen has a place to pool and won't be forced up and out. That also ensures that no air gets trapped to create a bubble which could split the condom. Roll the condom all the way to the base of your penis. Now you're ready for action. Put some water-based lubrication on the condom if needed. Immediately after ejaculation, hold the rim of the condom in place with a couple of fingers and withdraw your penis from her vagina while you still have an erection.

Use a fresh condom every time you have intercourse. Don't use snow-balling passion as an excuse to forget it a second or third time around. And for safety sake, use a condom for anal and oral sex too.

Finally, although the FDA has strict guidelines for condom manufacturing, some condoms break in use. The best way to avoid this is by using fresh ones. Check the expiration date on the package, and discard any over two years old because they may be brittle. Use only water-based lubricants; oil- and petroleum-based versions can degrade a condom and cause a break. Using a condom and spermicide (especially with an ingredient called nonoxynol-9) can further raise effectiveness against sexually transmitted diseases.

Store condoms properly away from heat (and tight confines of wallets). Check them after use. If you find a rupture, use spermicidal jelly or foam and talk to your doctor within two days about after-the-fact contraceptive options.

Get This: The classic complaint with condoms is loss of sensation (which, however, can be a blessing if you're interested in prolonging inter-

Emergency Contraception

If the worst happens, and you've engaged in unprotected sex, you can't undo the risk of sexually transmitted diseases. But you do have about 3 days to take action to prevent an unwanted pregnancy—assuming she agrees, of course, because obviously both methods concern her body.

Emergency contraception (EC) has been around since the 1960's, but not everyone knows about it, or how effective it can be. A "morning after pill" or an IUD inserted after the fact have both proven effective if your condom has broken, slipped, or you went ahead without one.[7] Minor side effects like nausea or headaches have been experienced, but can be treated with other medications. And don't depend on EC often; the methods lose effectiveness when used often. See a doctor or family planning office for details.

course). Two recent developments offer a solution which, not surprisingly, costs a little more. The first is an ultra thin latex version made by the Japanese. The second is non-latex condoms that are actually polyurethane, a material with two main advantages. First, you can safely use lubricants prohibited with latex, and, more dramatically, these newfangled ones are looser up top, so they allow the penis free movement inside. Get it? Penis movement. Friction. Suffice it to say there's a difference in sensation. Check it out.

Coitus interruptus

It certainly has a fancy name. Too bad coitus interruptus doesn't refer to a more valuable form of contraception. The act of withdrawing before orgasm is low in effectiveness for preventing pregnancy, and offers zero protection against STD's. That said, it's certainly better than nothing.

There are two major problems with coitus interruptus. First, it takes a lot of control to withdraw regularly before ejaculating. And even if you succeed, you may already be a couple of thrusts or even a few minutes too late: your penis sometimes releases a few drops of lubricating pre-ejaculatory fluid, which may contain sperm, especially if you've already had an orgasm.

Still, if amorous circumstances find you approaching orgasm and you haven't prepared in any way, coitus interruptus is much better than no contraception at all. But be prepared for extended time in the worry zone afterwards.

Effectiveness of coitus interruptus: an ineffective 20%.

Rhythm Method

The rhythm or "natural" method of contraception is based on the fact that a woman is able to conceive only one day or less every menstrual cycle. Avoid those hours and conception is avoided. The bad news is that it's hard to pinpoint that time, compounded by the fact that a man's sperm can live inside a woman for up to a week. So in order to maximize contraceptive efficiency with this method, intercourse should be avoided for a large block of time each month.

Because of religious or health concerns, some people won't use any other form of contraception. They need to know the fine points of estimating fertility, which demands serious observation, discipline, and patience. Using a calendar, a woman's temperature variations and vaginal mucus cycles, it's possible to estimate her fertility periods, and plan abstinence around them. Still, average contraceptive failure rates with the rhythm method are high, 20% or more. Plan to talk with a woman's health professional if you're seriously interested in this method. And as a man, be prepared for a limited window for intercourse. High discipline required.

Vasectomy

If you're sure you don't want children (or have enough already) and you're in a monogamous relationship (with no threat of STD's), a vasectomy just might be the perfect contraception for you. It's fairly simple as operations go. Sure, you have to get over the sound of "male sterilization." Maybe this outlook will help: spontaneous sex, day or night, all month long, with no more contraceptive devices or late periods to worry about.

Sounds good? You bet. Any drawbacks? Well, in theory a vasectomy is reversible only with a difficult and costly operation, with no guarantee of success. So be clear about your motivations in the first place.

Some men experience minor swelling and discomfort in one testicle, which may only last a week, but may continue for up to a year. And some research shows increased risk of prostate or testicular cancer in men with vasectomies. In one such study, reported in the Journal of the American Medical Association,[9] researchers found a link between

Go Figure

Of those reporting abstinence as their method of contraception, 26 percent become pregnant each year.[8]

prostate cancer and vasectomies, independent of other factors such as diet, exercise, and smoking. Another study found men with vasectomies to be 56% more likely to develop prostate cancer than those without.[10]

Those studies are disputed by others. In fact, the vast majority of doctors agree that more evidence would be needed for them to seriously question the procedure. Ultimately, you need to weigh the evidence and decide for yourself.

TAKE AN INSIDE LOOK

Physically, here's the story. Two tubes called the vas deferens carry sperm from the testicles to the urethra, which is the passageway running through the penis. After administering a local anesthetic, your doctor makes a small incision in the scrotum, cuts the tubes and either ties or cauterizes them closed. Some doctors now leave the testicle end open to reduce the possibility of swelling and pain some men experience. Sperm is still produced, it's simply absorbed by the body.

A new version of the operation is called the No-Scalpel Vasectomy. Instead of making a cut, the doctor punctures the skin and pulls the tubes out to cut and tie.

Either way, you're free to leave after the operation. After taking it easy for a couple of days to a week, you're ready to roll. It will take a few ejaculations to clear the tubes of sperm, so it's a good idea to have tests done to certify that the semen is sperm-free. After that, turn on the love lights.

COMING SOON TO A STORE OR LAB NEAR YOU?

Two new male contraceptive options loom in the future, although neither has yet achieved results which warrant breaking out the party hats.

First, an innovative practice combines the advantages of vasectomy with those of cryogenics. In short, a man would have his tubes tied after making a deposit in a sperm bank. He therefore prolongs his ability to father a child without worrying about the low rates of successfully reversing a vasectomy. Two researchers feel that this method represents a serious step forward in contraceptive practice, with technologies already present, and only widespread trials are needed to further widespread acceptance.[11]

The second has been on everyones lips for years, but unfortunately for those who are most interested, only figuratively speaking. It's the male birth control pill.

The good news is that finally there are genuine test results of a male pill. The bad news is that the results are mixed.[12]

The research followed eight Italian men who swallowed the two-hormone pills twice a day for 16 weeks. Four of the men showed a drop in sperm count to levels deemed by the World Health Organization to be officially infertile. William Bremner, the University of Washington researcher, noted that the problem was not all the men tested had success. So the ingredients and dosages need to be fine-tuned, but the results at least show that sperm counts can be lowered with a pill—a good starting point.

DESIRE

It's simple—*you want her.*

You're focused. Hot. Almost aching.

Sometimes sexual desire feels like a marching band, brassy and driven by drums. At other times it's a subtle awareness, like a breeze tickling curtains on a sultry summer evening. Either way, it's a good thing. Your pulse quickens, your skin flushes. First the touches are gentle, and soon bodies are heaving, moaning—the whole kit and caboodle.

But then again, it's not always so simple. This time you're not sure how much you want her. Or that time you clearly *didn't* want her—even as she lay beside you in lacy black panties that once made your heart thump.

While sex isn't all there is to a relationship, it can sure become a focal point when sexual desires don't match. The *Monogamy* chapter looks at desire in the context of relationships, including steps to keep it thriving. This chapter looks at *your* desire—what it is, and what to do when it's gone and you want it back.

LOOKING INTO DESIRE

Where does the erotic urge come from? Only in its absence do we really care. But then care we do, because it exerts a powerful pull even when absent. When we don't feel that wonderful erotic tug, that clarion call to action, we know we're missing something elemental, and we wonder why.

Sexual desire ebbs and flows naturally. A host of circumstances apply. Here we'll look at desire as a two-part phenomenon—a physical and a psychological event: first comes interest, and then a physical chain of events. But as Bernie Zilbergeld points out in *The New Male Sexuality*, we can wake up with an erection without any desire—it's good to realize that an erection and desire are not the same thing.[13] But when we become aware of something, whether a body, a scent, a memory, we're interested. When arousal follows interest, we're off and running. But what about when arousal doesn't follow, or you don't even feel the preliminary interest? Here are some common obstacles, followed by helpful tips for moving into the clear light of healthy sexual desire.

A CHECKLIST FOR OBSTACLES TO DESIRE

You'll find a range of desire blockers here (some with their own chapters in this book), which is no surprise since desire relates so directly to our over-all condition. This underscores our theme...

We're fortunate when just one factor is out of balance and easily cor-rected. But even when several factors are involved, a calm, level-headed approach will serve you best. Advances in knowledge and treatments of desire problems have led to solutions that work. But first, here are areas to consider when faced with low sexual desire.

Overall Health

First, don't panic. Sexual energy is one expression of your overall life ener-gy. Just as a couple's sex life expresses their overall relationship, your indi-vidual desire reflects your personal state of being. It's unrealistic to think that your sexual side should always have its own reservoir of ready energy. When our overall health is vital, it's fair to expect sexual vitality, but when we feel like we're firing on three cylinders, expecting instant sexual fire-works is folly. *Action step:* Evaluate your state of being. Ask your health provider for his or her opinion. Build your base level of well-being with proper nutrition and exercise. Lowered desire for sex may be an imporant wake-up call. So wake up!

Medications

Here is the most common culprit for low desire today. Many commonly pre-scribed drugs can lower libido. High blood pressure pills and antidepres-sants are popular and potentially desire-inhibiting examples. But there are many, many more. And there are no specific guidelines; everyone reacts to different medications differently. *Action step:* Talk to your doctor about changing your medication, lowering its dosage, or even not taking it for brief periods. He or she may have some simple answers you may not have considered. Consider natural alternatives, such as St. John's Wort for depres-sion, that don't generally affect sex drive. Bottom line: don't allow one phar-maceutical solution with available alternatives to rob you of the pleasure—and health-promoting nature—of sex.

Hormones

It's true: low testosterone levels in the bloodstream can cause low sexual desire. But, most experts agree, not in a large number of cases. Most typically the condition is found in older men. Replacing testosterone or other hormones such as DHEA has definitely boosted sex drive in some men. The generally accepted medical view recommends hormone replacement therapy only when tests have revealed low hormone levels. First, adding testosterone where levels are already normal doesn't add sexual desire or function, and it can lead to increased risk of prostate cancer or heart disease. *Action step:* Discuss testing for low hormones with your doctor. Simple saliva or blood tests are available.

Stress

Busy, busy, busy. Rush here, rush there, stand up, sit down—then have a profound sexual experience? Obviously something's wrong with that picture, and it's the incompatibility of satisfying sex and prolonged stress.

Okay, so stress is part of modern life, and to a degree a positive thing. But before rolling over and accepting its negative consequences, you need to ask yourself two questions: one, what is stress doing to me? And two, is it worth it? Stress can literally change your body's level of testosterone, the hormone associated with sexual desire.[14] Chronic stress is not just a hassle; it's a danger to your health, and a message that calls for a response. Impaired sexual function can indicate a life-threatening condition like heart disease. So sexual desire can be like the canary in a coal mine. Ignore its well-being at your peril. *Action step:* Read the *Stress* chapter. Take anti-stress action now. Learn how to relax. Make necessary lifestyle changes. Slow down and smell the roses. And her.

Expectations

Some men, and apparently some notable public figures, demand sex on a daily basis. For others, just a few times a month will do. A recent sex survey surprised many in its controversial revision of America's sex drive. The authors concluded that despite widespread assumptions to the contrary, Americans on average aren't as sexually active as many think.[15] Whether that study presents the absolute truth or not, it makes us realize that comparing ourselves to an imagined national desire quota is silly. The only proper standard of sexual frequency is our own satisfaction and that of our partner. But when one partner wants it more than the other, desire heats into a conflict that can devastate an otherwise happy relationship. *Action step:* Examine your expectations. Are they realistic? Adjust them if necessary, and don't allow the positive spirit of inquiry to dissolve into blame.

Depression

Depression is an increasingly common affliction in men. And a mood swing can easily banish your desire for sex. Antidepressant medication can boost a man's mood, but all too often it removes his desire for sex. New drugs show promise in that area, however. And for mild to moderate depression, the herb St. John's Wort has worked well for many men—with fewer and milder side effects and a lower cost. *Action step:* Ask your health care provider about the latest antidepressants. Many now recommend combining pharmaceutical medication with psychotherapy, which can go beyond fixing symptoms and get at the root of the problem. "Toughing out" depression is not the most efficient way to move beyond it. Exercise and nutrition changes should also be explored.

Anxiety

Being afraid is natural. Fear is a critical response that prepares us for danger. But when it becomes a general background state of being, that's anxiety, and it can easily destroy our desire for sex. Much of the preceding discussion of depression applies here. *Action step:* Medications and herbal remedies can help, as can exercise. Sometimes learning about sexual skills can help, or focusing less on intercourse. When you're less concerned about how sex will go, erotic impulses can flow more naturally. Developing communication skills is important. Trusting your inner voice enough to externalize it helps, as long as you're not trampling someone else's voice or desires. Psychotherapy can help develop your ability to feel, express, or defuse isolating emotions like anxiety, anger, and others discussed at length in the *Emotions* chapter.

EIGHT TIPS FOR RENEWING SEXUAL DESIRE

Having summarized common obstacles to desire, now we'll look at potent solutions for revitalizing a man's sex drive. Again, we'll start with physical options and move to the psychological.

Exercise

Low desire may simply be your body's way of telling you that it's time to get moving. A sedentary lifestyle is not what our bodies were designed for. And stress can compound the negative effects of the couch potato lifestyle. For the life of your cardiovascular, immune, skeletal, and sexual systems, just to name a few, start walking. Biking. Strength-training. Whatever rings your bell. Strength-training has reportedly boosted testosterone levels, which can supercharge desire for men at midlife or older. If you need help with finding the right exercise, consult your doctor or a personal fitness trainer.

Meditate

Meditation has moved out of Eastern monasteries. Now it's practiced even in Western hospitals, those bastions of high-tech, conventional medical care. Why? Because the health benefits have become clear. People start meditating for different reasons. Nourishing a sex drive might not be a common one, but it is one of the many benefits. That makes good common sense. Meditators often refer to their "practice." That practice is simply about being in the present, which sounds easy enough, until you try it. We spend so much time mentally rehashing the past or planning the future, it's surprising how little time we actually reside in the present. But sexual desire lives in the present. In time, meditation quiets the mind and allows you to be more receptive to subtle and not-so-sublte cues arising from within. Think of openness to internal sexual cues not as a goal of meditation, but as a byproduct. You can try it yourself with the simple instructions found in the *Stress* chapter.

Masturbate

Don't feel guilty about it. Whether you're in a sexual relationship or not, there are times when turning yourself on makes sense. Your genitals are built for use. Some doctors recommend moderate sexual activity for prostate health. So you owe it to your health, as well as your sexual desire, to experiment. If your day-to-day life isn't presenting sexual excitement, maybe you should create some. Spice things up. Try some pornography, or fantasize if you normally don't. Allow yourself the freedom to explore. It's certainly safer than cruising downtown for a prostitute. When stimulating yourself, spend some time focusing on the sensations. We'll come back to this in *Masturbation*, but for your own benefit, getting in touch with what feels good for you might be the first step in rediscovering your sexual spark.

Do Your Kegels

Speaking of sensations, kegel exercises not only strengthen your sex muscles, they can keep you in touch with them in a positive way (see the *Kegel Exercises* chapter if you don't know what they are). Bernie Zilbergeld, in *The New Male Sexuality*, offers an innovative way to use kegels to help with low desire.[16] The basic idea is to note when you find yourself being turned on in the course of an average day. You know, when the big-boned blond steps out of the elevator in a high-slit skirt? If you notice yourself having sexual thoughts, why not tune in on the sensations, and do a few kegels to acknowledge them? It's certainly not a move toward foolish sexual advances, just a way to keep in touch with your own sexuality, and keep in touch with it until you're in a position to appropriately express it with your sexual partner.

Try an Aphrodisiac

Again, not the ultimate long-term solution. But why not experiment to find something which might help light your fire? You might just make a discovery you wouldn't have otherwise considered. Oysters, for instance. With their high zinc content, they can boost all aspects of a man's sexuality, including desire. Or ginseng, whose sex-enhancing powers have been accepted in the Far East for centuries. Even pumpkin seeds: while not regarded as a great sex secret, they are rich in L-tryptophan, a precursor of the much-heralded, depression-busting serotonin,[17] which can help lift depression and the shadow it casts over sex.

Change your Attitude

That might sound like a broad suggstion, and it is. But you should consider if one or more attitudes is keeping you from accepting your natural sex drive. For instance, if you think you lack sexual skills, you should consider the validity of the judgment, whether self-imposed or received from a partner. Is is realistic? If so, can educating yourself help? This book and others offer solutions. A sex therapist can help, both with deciding if this is a problem or not, and with a number of helpful solutions. For example, how about a sex surrogate? It's an expensive option, but one that might be right for you. Working together with a psychologist, she can literally teach you how to make love. Of course, your normal sexual partner can do the same when good communication and trust are part of the relationship. Being willing to share, and able to trust, aren't always easy, but are worthy of pursuing for long-term sexual desire and satisfaction.

Use Contraception

Fear of pregnancy can take the sizzle out of sex, or prevent it altogether. But proper contraception, consciously practiced, is a blue ribbon solution. With a range of contraceptive options available for men and women, it's easy to find one that's right for you. Of course, most do carry small risks of pregnancy, so if even those chances are too great, you might consider sexual alternatives to intercourse.

Contraceptives such as condoms or diaphragms needn't interfere with the spontaneity of sex. Feeling too uncomfortable to stop and start, or talk and laugh, is a sign of needless tension. Remember, in many ways sex is about relaxing and enjoying the flow. Sure, there's a tension involved, but it should be a background motivation more than what happens front and center. Again, communication can make all the difference. Many men can profit from learning better communication skills, which help in many ways, including, in this case, not letting contraceptives interfere with the natural upwelling of desire for sex.

See a Therapist

For a man raised in this country at this time, some relationship skills like feeling and expressing emotions don't come easy. But we don't have to feel threatened by them. No one is suggesting that a man give up his masculinity. Fortunately, the old stereotype of the tall, dark, and silent male hero is losing its appeal. One very good reason for that is studies which tell us that isolating ourselves and holding in some emotions can be harmful to our health, leading to heart disease, depression and other places we'd prefer not to visit. The problem, of course, is that some habits are hard to change, even in a close and loving relationship. That's where sex therapy, or psychotherapy, can help. Therapists are trained to help in these areas. It's not hard to tell when one is needed. Emotional pain and suffering often precede the decision to explore this option. If you just don't feel a sexual spark and your doctor can't find a reason, try a therapist. Ask friends for referrals, or call a local psychological association.

EJACULATION

It's beautiful! Not only is ejaculation the perfect sperm delivery system, the grand finale of male sexuality, speeding millions of tiny encoded versions of yourself toward their destiny; it feels great too!

But more precisely, while ejaculation sends forth semen, orgasm precedes it and produces the ecstasy. Exploring that difference leads into one of the hottest, most promising area of male sexuality today, and it also touches on one of the most troubling.

By separating orgasm from ejaculation, more and more men are prolonging their pleasure, having more intense orgasms, and enjoying multiple orgasms. And by lengthening the time from arousal to ejaculation, many men troubled by premature ejaculation are finding new satisfaction in sex.

All of which we'll explore now.

THE ANATOMY OF COMING

In order to put ejaculation in perspective, here's the story of semen in a nutshell. Produced in the testicles, sperm moves into the epididymis tubes, directly behind each testicle, where it grows until ready to wriggle up the vas deferens tubes to where the tubes widen into a staging area near the prostate gland. Here sperm will be mixed with fluids from the prostate gland and seminal vesicles, which nourish and condition the sperm for its journey ahead. At this point we have semen, not just sperm.

Now, some will object to comparing the penis to a gun, but the analogy certainly works for ejaculation. Just prior to ejaculation, the semen moves into the urethra (the tube that extends from the bladder and prostate to the end of the penis), as if a bullet into a chamber. Nerve impulses arrive at the pelvic floor, or PC, muscles, which contract rhythmically and forcefully, and send the semen on its merry way. Boom—ejaculation.

JUMPING THE GUN

Although that analysis sounds simple in theory, ejaculation often goes wrong, or more accurately, happens too soon, in premature or rapid ejaculation, which one male sexuality expert estimates as affecting one third of

American men.[18] Unlike erectile dysfunction, which the medical profession now regards as mostly physiologically-based, premature ejaculation is considered to be mainly psychological in nature—not so much based in emotions, though, as simply undeveloped awareness of the full range of sensations between arousal and orgasm. For various reasons, many men learn early in their lives to rush to orgasm. Maybe it was the hurried masturbation to avoid being caught, or the need to be quick to avoid the policeman's flashlight at lovers lane, or just good old insecurity in early sexual relationships when orgasm was the only goal. The good news is rapid ejaculation, since it was learned, can be unlearned too, with steps that men can learn and practice alone or with a sexual partner.

So how fast is too fast? In the past, supposedly objective criterion prevailed, such as how many minutes, how many thrusts, etc. Now new definitions have emerged: rapid ejaculation is frequently coming before (or quickly after starting) intercourse; or simply sooner than either partner would like. That last phrase is key.

Sex resists objective standards. What is too quick in one relationship is perfectly fine in another. There's a good lesson there: judge yourself, if judge you must, not by what your buddy says, or this video or that book, but what works well for you and your partner. Find what's true for you by knowing your own heart and hers. Once again, that means openness. Communication. A willingness to listen. When ejaculation in that context is too soon, not only are proven solutions available, but they will more likely be effective, because having a partner who's engaged in the process will help.

SLOWING DOWN

It's important to put rapid ejaculation in perspective. Prolonging the time between arousal and ejaculation is a relatively recent goal, and unique to the human species. While animals lavish much energy on extravagant courtship displays, sex itself takes just seconds.[19] Men are exploring new territory here, which is one reason why a definition of rapid ejaculation is so hard to establish. One estimate of the average elapsed time from start of arousal to male climax is three minutes.[20] Should we think of that as a reasonable goal, too fast, or what?

Averages aside, a man doesn't need a definition to know what's too fast. It's something felt, either in him or his partner, and he's often all too familiar with the accompanying feelings: frustration, anger, anxiety, and low self-esteem, for starters, and the familiar stress they produce. But it's equally important to keep in mind that these emotions are not broadly considered to be the cause of rapid ejaculation, but reactions to it—an important distinction. The most commonly accepted cause is moving from arousal to ejaculation *automatically*, without really feeling the sensations in between. Getting in touch with those sensations is the road on which many man have traveled back to more satisfying sex lives. We'll look at time-tested techniques for doing just that.

But first, here are a few solutions most of us have heard about at one time or another: a quick, private orgasm in the bathroom before sex with a partner; using one, two, or more condoms; multiplication tables or other mental distractions recited during intercourse; and imbibing alcohol beforehand. The problem with those is that even if they work (and they can), they can mean less involvement in the act itself. Even if the battle is won, the quality of the victory is questionable.

Some men want the problem to disappear by taking a pill; some doctors will oblige, and that can work too. The hidden risk, with antidepressants or other pharmaceutical solutions to premature ejaculation, comes in the form of side effects. For some, they're worth it; for others, not.

EIGHT STEPS TO SLOW EJACULATION

If you're frequently ejaculating too soon, you probably want a quick answer to the problem. That's natural. But when slowing ejaculation is the goal, slowing down in general is the starting point.

You can last longer by becoming more aware of the full range of sexual sensations, which will take some time, but will be well worth the effort. Consider not rushing to intercourse, or even partnered sex. In fact, the most popular techniques to slow ejaculation are found on a continuum between stimulating yourself and learning to last longer during intercourse. Here are a few steps along the way.

Masturbate

Self-pleasuring can help you become more aware of all sensations, physical and emotional, beginning with arousal. You'll find details and fine points in the *Masturbation* chapter. But here's a goal: learning to stimulate yourself for 15 minutes before coming. The timing, of course, isn't cast in stone, but

15 minutes is a generally accepted threshold for the ability to have more control. Of course your emphasis should be on sensations, not watching the clock. Start with a shorter length of time. Try longer. Exploration is the key. Stroke, squeeze, hold, whatever feels good—the point is only to feel it all. Feel the acceleration of arousal, the approach to the point of inevitability, of not being able to stop anymore, and ejaculation itself. This is not self-indulgence. For many it's the very basis for having more control when with a partner.

Do Kegels

These exercises also have their own chapter. But they're important in this context because they can help develop awareness of the physical sensations of ejaculation, as well as developing muscular control which will help. In fact, learning kegel exercises can be the first time a man becomes conscious of the existence and location of muscles producing ejaculation. As we'll see in *Taoist Sex*, developing these muscles provides dividends that go well beyond restoring a more satisfying ejaculation time. It enables a man to develop the ability to expand lovemaking profoundly, including whole-body and multiple orgasms.

Think Love

This is an important shift that not only helps a man to last longer, but can revolutionize his approach to sex. Mantak Chia, author of *The Multi-Orgasmic Man*, says that sex magnifies whatever emotions you feel, and negative emotions can limit your ability to control your ejaculation.[21] His Taoist tradition stresses the energetic connection of genitals and heart, which meshes easily with the less esoteric revelations of common sense. You know that the physical, mental, and emotional state of love and caring are much different, and much preferable for satisfying sex, than the stress-related states of anger, anxiety, nervousness, or impatience. So to last longer, make love, not war.

Don't Forget to Breathe

Breathing is an important link between bodily processes you can control and those you can't. You can't stop it voluntarily, but you can change *how* you breathe.

Various breathing exercises are commonly used to relax and center, and can be used to slow ejaculation. Slow, deep breathing works for some, while shallow rapid breathing works for others. Synchronized breathing can deepen your connection to your lover. More on that in *Tantric Sex*.

Try Polarity Sex

This is a fancy name for a simple approach: First one partner concentrates on bringing his or her partner to orgasm, then that partner reciprocates. This is a basic formula for many couples. For a man, it might mean lengthening foreplay and bringing his lover to orgasm before intercourse. Since most women require more time than men to climax, and many don't have vaginal orgasms, this approach is natural and appreciated. And it takes the pressure off a man to prolong ejaculation. Feeling more relaxed, he can better stay with the sensations and emotions of sex.

Stop and Start

This is the first of two classic techniques that have helped many men. The Stop/Start approach was developed in this country by a urologist named Dr. James Semans in the fifties. It uses the whole range from self-pleasuring to partnered sex.[22] The technique is useful to men marginally affected by rapid ejaculation and those with the more acute problem of coming even before intercourse begins. A few weeks of practice should make a substantial difference in your ability to last longer.

Again, the goal—and the process—is to relax, to be more present for what's happening. So right from the start, be more aware of what you feel when masturbating, without lubrication. The point is to stimulate yourself until you feel the approach of ejaculation. Then stop. Relax. Feel the sensations. Find what works best for you, either letting go of your penis or holding without stroking. When you feel the urge to ejaculate recede, begin again. Try doing this for 15 minutes without coming. If you move past the point of no return and ejaculate, don't worry about it. That's why you're doing

---

Stop/Start Bonus

As part of the stop/start process, pay attention to what your whole body is feeling, not just your penis. Sexual arousal felt throughout the body can increase the intensity of your orgasms.[23]

this exercise. Just try it again when you're ready.

Next, try using lotion, still while self-pleasuring. This tends to intensify the sensations and can make stopping more challenging. When you're ready, the next step is not to stop when you feel the approach of inevitability, but vary

> **Did You Know?**
>
> Rapid ejaculation is hardest to control in the classic man-on-top missionary position. Less muscular exertion is needed for (and less tension results from) the woman being on top.

your stimulation in terms of pressure and stroke. Again, try for 15 minutes, and don't be surprised if you ejaculate in spite of your best efforts. It's all good practice, and part of getting where you want to go.

When you feel confident about controlling ejaculation by yourself, then it's time to get your partner involved. The steps are basically the same: dry masturbation, wet masturbation (or oral sex), with stop/vary instead of stop/start. Then you're ready to use the techniques during intercourse, first stopping, then varying movements, thrusts, and positions. Optimal relaxation is enhanced by good communication with your partner throughout this process. If you need more help during the intercourse phase, try the next technique.

Squeeze

This technique shares similarities with the stop/start approach. But instead of stopping stimulation of the penis, this technique is more aggressive: first in masturbation, and then with intercourse, when a man approaches the point of no return, the woman stops and squeezes his penis until his arousal decreases to the point where he can start again.

Her thumb, or thumbs in the two-handed version, should be on the frenulum of his penis (just below the head on the underside); her first finger should rest on the other (top) side of his penis with her other fingers below it on the shaft. The pressure should be firm but obviously not too much so. When he signals, either by an agreed-upon signal or verbally, that he is ready to continue, she resumes either manual stimulation or with intercourse.

Both of these last two techniques can be practiced up to three times a week for several weeks. If no positive changes result in that time, ask your doctor about alternatives.

Hug Until Relaxed

David Schnarch, author of the groundbreaking book *Passionate Couples*, offers an interesting solution to interpersonal tension that can help rapid ejaculation.[24] His prescription is to hug until both partners feel themselves relax. The technique is not about relaxing the other person. He doesn't present this as a solution per se for rapid ejaculation, but one that helps relieve tension and offers a good starting point for sex.

EJACULATION IN THE WORLD

Ted was a college junior when a noted sex therapist spoke to a packed assembly in his school's gymnasium. Some of the more conservative professors in the audience were shocked, but judging by the many detailed questions, the students were not. The sex expert mentioned several techniques for slowing ejaculation.

Ted had lost his virginity only two years before and had been embarrassed by rapid ejaculation in both of his romantic relationships since then. He couldn't last more than a few seconds during intercourse.

As Ted sat with Donna, his girlfriend, in the audience that day, he felt uncomfortable and grateful at the same time. He was happy to hear several new ways to help with his problem. He knew he could last as long as he wanted while masturbating, and was thankful that Donna was understanding and willing to help.

The next time they slept together, he suggested the squeeze technique, but she felt too self-conscious doing it. Then they tried stopping and starting instead, which worked better, although the first few times he still came sooner than he liked. In three weeks he found he didn't have to stop altogether. Instead he moved in a circular direction inside her as an alternative to thrusting. Another friend suggested keeping his butt muscles relaxed. That helped too. But things really improved when Donna was on top. Over time, their sex improved to the point where Ted still liked her on top; he held her hips to keep her from moving too wildly when she got fully aroused.

EMOTIONS

Be happy more, and angry less. Enjoy good health longer. Prosper at work. Develop deep, lasting relationships, *and supercharge your sex life!* It's all possible by exploring the world of emotions—your emotions.

For too long, too many men have been emotional black holes. Independent, strong, and silent, but also angry, anxious, or depressed, and enjoying less sex than they care to admit.

Nor is feeling numb new for men. But while that's not good news, neither is it the end of the world. In fact, the vague awareness that your life is missing something is critical, because it's the vital first step in the revitalizing process of renewal.

Why now? Why you? Hey, the world is changing. And so is a man's place in it, with different demands at work, around the house, and in committed relationships.

The good news is that every man has a strong, built-in system of stabilizing cues, messages that appear involuntarily to warn or motivate. They're called emotions. It's time to stop thinking about them as good or bad. Time to forget about your head in opposition to your heart. It's time to tune into your emotions and appreciate their power to lead you to intimacy, deep satisfaction, and lasting confidence.

In this chapter, we'll take a close look at emotions. What they are. Why men avoid them. And why there is no optimum sexual fitness in today's world when they are ignored.

JUST FEEL IT

One simple question leads you into the rewarding realm of emotion: what are you feeling?

What are you feeling? Far too many men can't answer that question. Try as they may, they just can't find the words. Or even feel the feelings. Sound confusing? Well it doesn't have to be. In fact, with a sustained effort, every man can tune into his feelings—and be surprised by how much they enrich his life. Does this mean surrendering your manhood? Absolutely not! Nowhere is it written that in silence is strength, or in avoidance of strong feelings, success. On the contrary, much has already been written, with much yet to come, about the incredible benefits of acknowledging your emotions and integrating them into your day-to-day existence at work and home.

Let's begin with a word so new it's probably not in your dictionary. Alexithymia—the inability to name one's own emotions. In other words, emotional illiteracy. That's right—many men can read and write fine but when it comes to describing their own feelings they're in the dark. Of course that sets them on a collision course with women, who from childhood have been hunkered down with friends, exploring the ins and outs of hundreds of feelings. So men and women often have very different orientations to feeling. Often that difference simmers on the back burner, but where sex is concerned it heats up considerably. Often to the point of boiling.

So what are these things called emotions that bring us such discomfort—and pleasure?

Every emotion is a physiological event, a reaction in your body to some stimulus in the inner or outer world. In his groundbreaking book, *Emotional Intelligence*, Daniel Goldman notes that every emotion is "an impulse to act."[25]

Think about that. When we feel anger, fear, or love, for instance, things happen in our body, and those impulses prepare us—through the intricate and lightning-fast reactions of hormonal chemistry—to *do* something. That's where emotions as messages comes into play, and where the value of emotions lies. They're alerting you to pay attention to movement in the dark. Advising you about how to handle a sticky situation at work, and urging you to approach, or at times avoid, that mysterious creature called your girlfriend or wife.

But before we can learn to let our emotions help us, we need to tune into them as they occur. Learn to feel them. Appreciate them. The best way to do that is to develop our emotional literacy.

JUST LABEL IT

In *Passion and Reason*, Richard and Bernice Lazarus wisely advance the idea that thinking and feeling aren't opposed to one another. In fact their book proceeds from the idea that every emotion has a purpose—in each moment and in the larger view of each individual's values.

We've noted that paying attention to emotions is the first step in gaining control over them, which is important for those that keep us from intimate connection with a lover.

Now let's look beyond the all-too-common, black or white labeling of emotions as good or bad. As we explore our emotional lives, we find valuable surprises.

We are a constant play of emotions. Though feelings of anger, fear, or happiness are the most obvious, there are many, many more happening whether we're aware of them or not. Need examples? Well for starters:[26]

abandoned	competitive	fearful
addicted	confused	flustered
adequate	crazy	foolish
affectionate	cruel	free
agitated	crushed	frightened
ambivalent	daring	frustrated
amused	deceitful	frivolous
annoyed	defeated	furious
anxious	delighted	gallant
apathetic	desirous	glad
arrogant	despairing	gloomy
ashamed	determined	good
astonished	diminished	graceful
awed	discontented	gratified
bashful	distracted	greedy
betrayed	disturbed	grieving
bitter	divided	groovy
blissful	dominated	guilty
blue	eager	gullible
bold	ecstatic	happy
bored	edgy	hateful
brave	electrified	helpful
calm	empty	helpless
capable	enchanted	high
challenged	energetic	homesick
charmed	envious	honored
cheated	exasperated	horny
cheerful	excited	horrible
childish	exhausted	hurt
clever	exuberant	hysterical
combative	fascinated	ignored

immortal
impressed
indifferent
infatuated
infuriated
insecure
inspired
intimidated
intolerant
isolated
jealous
jilted
jittery
joyous
kind
kinky
lazy
lecherous
lonely
low
lucky
mad
mean
melancholic
miserable
mocked
moody
mournful
mystical
nasty
nervous
nice
numb
obnoxious
obsessed

obstinate
odd
offended
opposed
ornery
outraged
overlooked
panicked
peaceful
persecuted
petrified
pitiful
pleasant
pleased
poetic
pressured
proud
pushy
quarrelsome
quirky
refreshed
rejected
rejuvenated
relaxed
relieved
reluctant
remorseful
restless
reverent
rewarded
righteous
robust
sad
satisfied
scared

secure
sexy
silly
sneaky
solemn
sorrowful
spiteful
sympathetic
talkative
tempted
tender
tense
tentative
terrible
terrified
threatened
thwarted
trapped
troubled
ugly
uneasy
unsettled
upset
vain
violent
vulnerable
wicked
wired
wistful
weepy
wonderful
woozy
worried
zoned out

But hey, you're not an emotional guy, right? So why are words from that list so familiar? The point is simply this: emotions fill our day-to-day lives. Sure, there are plenty of circumstances when it's just not appropriate to express them. In fact, one theory holds that man, historically the hunter and warrior, lived with courser emotions when his days were filled with split-second, live-or-die reactions. But that changed radically when your adversary is a business colleague that uses indirect, emotionally-loaded half-truths to advance his standing and hurt yours. Or when your lover wants to know how you feel about her making more money than you. Or her asking to move your shared sex out of its rut. Man, then it's time to step up. Open up. Recognize your feelings, and be willing and able to talk about them, and act on them appropriately.

CONNECTING SEX WITH FEELINGS

So what's the sexual benefit in all this? Not much if all you're interested in is a quick fuck with a stranger. But the moment you get involved in a relationship, and specifically a sexual relationship, your emotional involvement determines where the relationship goes. Or doesn't go.

Dr. Ronald Levant, author of *Masculinity Reconstructed*, refers often to what he calls unconnected lust.[27] He notes that most men are conditioned from early childhood to be goal-oriented and emotionally inexpressive. So by the time boy becomes man, his need for closeness and intimacy is in conflict with and subservient to his need to achieve. Therefore his sex drive, his physical lust, often remains unconnected with his needs for intimacy and love. And as we've already noted, that produces a one-dimensional relationship. Without intimacy, sex moves away from shared satisfaction and becomes a one-sided list of demands. On one hand, it means a man making love with a woman; on the other, a man having sex with a bra, or with a fantasy instead of a person. Being sexually fit, being the best a man can be, means being able to share tenderness, be intimate, make love. The smart man learns how emotions can lead him there and make him whole. Be patient, because emotions are intimately entwined with the big lessons of your life, which never end. Becoming a man, as Hemingway wrote, takes a lifetime.

BE A MAN—BE RESPONSIBLE

Psychologists use the word projection, to refer to sending emotions outward that are too uncomfortable to accept inwardly—in other words, not taking responsibility for one's own emotions. Someone else is making you angry, frustrated, depressed. Always someone else. It must be their fault. And so on, as they say in Latin, ad nauseum.

Sometimes accepting responsibility is tough. Especially for messy, unpleasant emotions. But the reward is well worth the effort. You feel new freedom. Enjoy new power. Become a better partner. But it takes effort. Win a multimillion dollar contract? Build a house by yourself? Incredible achievements, surely, but not greater achievements than taking responsibility for your own emotions.

FIVE EMOTIONS AND SEXUAL FITNESS

Emotions play a major part in determining the quality of your life, and sex life. Learn how to recognize them, control them if desired (and possible), live with them, and value them. Because they're so common, and so important, we'll take a close look at a few of the most powerful.

Anger

Possibly the most energetic of emotions, anger can get you into a heap of trouble fast, and can do lasting damage to a sexual relationship. The jury is still out on exactly how damaging it is to your health, but evidence is mounting. In one study of men with previous heart attacks, those who were easily angered were three times more likely to die of heart failure.[28] And anger is known to render you more vulnerable to a range of less severe health problems.[29]

More often than not, anger arises in response to a real or perceived attack.[30] We feel threatened, and react defensively, hoping to protect or restore our well-being.

Once aroused, anger flares and spreads like a brush fire. It's fed by combustible thought patterns, can change direction easily, and can do major irreparable damage. It's a sure damper of sexual desire, incompatible with the subtler perceptions and connections necessary for its flowering. And of course, anger easily creates emotional and physical barriers which rule out sex altogether.

Rage, irritation, bitterness, etc.—it comes in many forms, all with nasty consequences. Often the first step in controlling anger is the hardest: recognizing it. Since anger is often fueled by stress biochemicals, we're not

Seven Tips for Dealing with Anger

- *Get away.* The most immediate step to stop the flow of stress hormones is physically removing yourself from the object of your anger. Having an intense argument with your lover and it's just spiraling downward out of control? Take a time out. Do some jumping jacks on the lawn. Go for a walk around the block. If this is not possible, counting to ten or deep breathing can help break your focus on the dance of anger.

- *Feel it out.* The heroic inner response to anger is not to immediately send it out into the world. In war, possibly, but in the context of a sexual relationship, no. It's yours—feel it, explore it, and profit from it. Otherwise you're just staying on a treadmill, and endlessly repeating a loop of destructive energy.

- *Go beyond blowing off steam.* Okay, sometimes jabbing at a punching bag feels like the perfect response. But while it may be an effective safety valve, your anger may disappear but it merely goes underground, without being resolved, with the same response ready to rear its ugly head another time.

- *Don't let it fester.* The time to talk about some things is when they happen. Talk to your lover about what bothers you when you react to it, not after weeks of stewing in angry resentment. It may feel uncomfortable to air your feelings right away, but not nearly like after waiting too long.

- *Keep angry words focused.* When you're able to talk and not shout, tell your lover what you feel and think about the subject at hand. Throwing in assorted, unrelated frustrations will only fan the fire. You might think you're gaining something by adding more artillery, but you're only prolonging the conflict and making it more painful.

- *Share what you're feeling, not blame.* Anger is a strong reaction. As soon as you can, and hopefully right from the start, use it to convey what you feel about something. This is the critical first step in taking responsibility for your own emotions. And the best way to transform two shouting heads into connected lovers. Try "It makes me feel ____ when you do ___, " instead of the inflammatory and non-productive, "You're a ____ for doing ___."

- *Don't say things you'll regret.* Everyone knows how it feels to have said something needlessly hurtful and then wish you hadn't. Some things can't be forgotten. The only way for them not to be in your lover's mind is not to say them in the first place.

primed to think, we're prepared for action. And most of us have familiar anger responses ready to feed the flame. Even when we see it developing, it's difficult to stop.

But the more we're objective about anger's damage, and able to look at our role in it, the more incentive we have to control it, or certainly to minimize it's impact.

Depression

Depression can feel like no emotion at all. Or a mix of emotions, such as anger (turned inward), grief, dejection, and/or hopelessness. Symptoms range from exhaustion, irritability, enjoying friends less, problems concentrating, to brooding about death.

One in ten American men will have at least one serious bout of depression in his lifetime.[31] And untreated, many of those will experience its symptoms, including loss of sexual desire and ability, on a chronic basis. Add the classic male response of denying health problems, and you have a recipe for trouble. Which is reflected in the fact that 23,000 American men commit suicide every year.[32]

The good news is that tremendous advances have been made in treating this widespread affliction. Antidepressant medication such as Prozac, Zoloft, Wellbutrin and others have successfully lifted moods for millions of Americans of both sexes. But even the most popular, Prozac, works for only approximately 6 in 10 of those who try it.[33] And then there's the much-publicized loss of libido and other side effects. They have motivated some to try natural alternatives, which have successfully treated mild to moderate cases of depression, with fewer and milder side effects.

Is our society becoming a more depressing place? That's a question everyone has to answer for himself, but for those experiencing symptoms of depression, the more pressing question is how to help themselves feel better.

Anxiety

Fear can spread over time, lose its connection to a specific cause, and become a broad, underlying state of being. When this happens it is anxiety, which can also manifest itself in a range of obsessions and phobias. We're uneasy, worried, up tight, and in the extreme, feel panic, causing such symptoms as increased sweating, a dry mouth, headaches, and irregular heartbeat. Sexually, anxiety casts its wide shadow over everything from

Five Tips for Beating the Blues

- *Exercise.* Millions successfully use exercise to beat stress, get energized, and boost moods. Walking, jogging, swimming, strength-training, among many others, can make you look and feel better naturally. See the *Exercise* chapter for details.
- *Change your diet.* There are many ways to understand depression, and one is biochemistry. The miracle of healthy brain function depends on nerve cells and chemicals such as serotonin and dopamine which transmit messages. The famous antidepressants of the last decade—selective serotonin reuptake inhibitors (SSRIs) like Prozac and Paxil—boost the serotonin-induced sense of well-being. Similarly, a number of vitamins and minerals in foods work to ensure an optimum supply of those same brain chemicals.[34] B vitamins, Vitamin C, Selenium, and their sources like leafy greens, fish, and whole grains are just a few of the phytonutrients (plant nutrients) known to influence mood in some people. If you're depressed, simple dietary changes may be a smart first choice in healing.
- *Reach out.* Many studies now show that having a social support system encourages good health, and it can be critical in balancing downward-spiraling depressed thoughts. Men especially tend to isolate themselves rather than seek the help of friends or doctors. And seeking solace in drugs or alcohol not only doesn't help the depression, it keeps the problem hidden, contributing to what many call a growing, silent epidemic of depression. Don't be part of it. Reach out to your lover, friends, family, or your doctor, and get back on track.
- *See a therapist.* Contrary to what too many men feel, there's no shame in seeing a psychologist. In fact, it may be the most efficient way to explore counterproductive attitudes, emotions, and behaviors. All of us were conditioned in childhood to see and act and feel in some counterproductive ways; the intimacy of sex can bring them to the forefront, causing rocky relationships and plunging spirits. A therapist is a specialist who can help you identify and move past emotions and attitudes that are holding you back. A good therapist doesn't dispense answers, he or she teaches you to ask the right questions, and find your own solutions.
- *Consider an antidepressant.* When you can't pull your spirits up on your own, and it's interfering with your work and relationships, talk to your therapist or doctor about available medications. A range of antidepressants can help. And you don't have to trade your sex life to take them. Ask your doctor about substituting one drug for another, reducing the dosage, or taking short breaks from the medication, which boosts desire without interfering with the drug's mood-lifting power. Or talk to an alternative health provider about herbs and other natural treatments that minimize the side effects, such as St. John's Wort or the Ayurvedic herb ashwagandha. And there's exciting news for those interested in combining the best of both conventional and natural medicines. A study published in the *Journal of Sex & Marital Therapy* showed the herb ginkgo biloba 84% effective in counteracting sexual problems caused by SSRI antidepressant medications.[35]

Four Steps for Easing Anxiety

- *De-stress yourself.* Since anxiety is a big part of stress, stress reduction can reduce anxiety. Both can be anchored in an imagined threat, and fueled by stress hormones flooding your system, preparing you to act in response to danger. Even if the danger is based in the past, as with sexual problems, or focused on the future, like general financial worries, the physical response is real and in the present. The appropriate response is to take action. Exercise is a powerful coping strategy. Others are detailed in the *Stress* chapter. The important thing is to start the counter-stress responses your mind and body are equipped with to override dangerous inner stress reactions in even the most outwardly serene lives.

- *Think differently.* One branch of psychology, the cognitive approach, says you can change your behavior by changing your thinking. In this case, your behavior is worrying with such intensity or frequency that your body readies itself for danger, which creates an enlarging loop of worry. Break that cycle by creating an opposing, and positive, picture. Tell yourself you can do so-and-so. Create the reality you want. Changing how you think about a problem can be a giant step toward finding a good solution. Learning to observe and counteract anxious thoughts can help shift you away from anxiety toward worry-free relief.

- *Meditate.* Learning to function more in the present and less in an anxiety-ridden past or future is a powerful benefit of meditation. As detailed in the *Stress* chapter, meditating can promote health by reversing the stress response. It can help you be more aware of anxiety-producing thoughts as they begin to arise. And it can make you more receptive to what's happening in the present, like your lover beckoning.

- *Seek help.* When none of the above help, it's time to ask a health provider and/or psychotherapist for help. Medications can smooth out anxiety, helping you to get on with your life. As with medications for depression, some of which are used for anxiety, they offer powerful results but can bring unwanted side effects, including problems with sexual desire and performance. And again, natural alternatives like the herbs Kava Kava, Skullcap, and St. John's Wort have brought relief to many without the side effects, and at lower costs. Ask your doctor or a certified herbalist to explain the risks and benefits.

desire to performance to self-image. Maurice Yaffé and Elizabeth Fenwick, authors of *Sexual Happiness for Men*, even refer to relationship anxiety,[36] where a man questions his ability for intimacy with a woman altogether.

Like depression, anxiety can gradually over-influence your mental and emotional life, leaving you less able to function smoothly and efficiently at home and work. But as with depression, there are several steps you can take to take back control of your life.

Jealousy

It's all over the woman-to-woman grapevine: if you're uncomfortable with a man's jealousy, *leave the relationship as quickly as possible!* Now that's serious advice! Why so? To find out, let's back up a moment and define jealousy.

Possibly no other emotion feels so much like one thing but is in fact something else. Jealousy might feel like love, like caring and attention. But too often it's an expression of fear and slumping self-esteem, which too often produce very negative consequences. It gets back to the projection dynamic mentioned earlier. A man might think a woman is untrustworthy, but it's really his inability to trust. What might start out as simple jealous remarks can rapidly decay into picking out her clothes, determining what friends she can see, isolating her, and finally, in the ultimate relationship toxicity, abusing her.

Of course, it's not always that extreme. Most men feel twinges of jealousy now and again. Some female flirting (like the male version) is reasonably problematic. But feeling a twinge of jealousy is very different from battering a woman. If you or anyone you know is unsure of the ability to stop the slide from one to the other, encourage professional help. Fast. Of the 3-4 million women battered every year, 2 million are seriously injured.[37] That's a serious mark against American manhood.

Like anger, to which it's related and often feeds, jealousy is hard to control, especially because it so distorts a man's judgment. Question it. Never act foolishly under its influence. And if it approaches the irreversible option of abuse, seek help immediately.

Happiness

Thomas Jefferson made it a fundamental right of all Americans. The Dali Lama calls it "the very purpose of your life."[38] And you certainly like it when you feel it. So why does happiness sometimes seem so hard to find, and hold on to, and how does sex fit in?

Psychology has focused on unhappiness and how to alleviate it, but has said surprisingly little about happiness and how to achieve it. So we're left on our own to figure out the path to well-being, contentment, satisfaction, cheerfulness, and ecstasy. Richard and Bernice Lazarus make an interesting distinction n their book *Passion and Reason*. They see well-being as a background condition while happiness is an emotion that comes and goes in the foreground.[39] Whether we're happy at any given time depends to some extent on how we are overall, our sense of well-being. This applies to our sex life in an interesting way.

Judging by tales of sex heard on the ball field or in a bar, you'd think that individual "scores," or acts of sex constitute sexual satisfaction. But anyone in a lasting relationship knows better. In time, the gaudy and randy newness of sex is bound to fade. And then a man faces a choice: scuttle off to greener pastures, or find the courage to look within, commit, and contribute to a mature sexual relationship, whether it lasts three years or a lifetime.

Mature men know that great sex is a matter of shared intimacy, which takes time and trust to build. Despite the inevitable ups and downs, that's true sexual happiness and well-being.

EMOTION IN THE WORLD

Jeff remembers the specific moment his marriage changed forever, and for better.

It had been a typical argument with Ann. She had complained again about his not helping enough with their children. True, Jeff's business travel had been taking him away more than usual. But he had also been making a real effort to help out around the house lately, and had just taken the kids downtown for the whole afternoon, which is why her complaint seemed so unfounded. He suspected she was feeling frustrated again about not working. She liked being a full-time mom but did miss the intensity of her former work as an attorney.

Jeff knew all that and couldn't stop the argument from escalating into a classic shouting match. But then he remembered something he and his therapist had been discussing: withdrawing projections. When that thought crossed his mind he went into the spare bedroom of the house they were temporarily renting and closed the door. He lay down on the floor, in the orange shag carpet. He felt the anger, the intense energy in his chest.

As he lay there, he consciously stopped blaming Ann for how he was feeling. He consciously pulled his anger back, took possession of it, and accepted it as his own. The amazing thing was, as he lay there almost physically pulling the anger back, he felt it intensely—and then it faded. Later, when he went out to talk with Ann, she could tell something was different. She didn't know what, but her anger drained away too.

Jeff had made an incredible discovery. By tuning into his anger instead of hurling it out, he assumed responsibility for it. He owned it. That felt deeply right. And as he has continued to do it (sometimes with more success than others), he knows it has made him and his marriage stronger.

EXERCISE

American males fall into two categories. Those who exercise and those who don't.

If you're among the latter, listen up: inactive lifestyles account for five times as many American deaths as car accidents.[40] To put that in perspective, it's roughly five times the American fatalities in the Vietnam War.

If you already exercise regularly, you probably already enjoy the extraordinary benefits, such as:

- looking good—being literally more attractive to the ladies
- keeping your weight where you want it
- boosting your energy
- building stamina
- staying healthy
- neutralizing stress
- remaining supple

Which of these isn't a plus for your sex life?

Plus, there's that mysterious feeling of well-being associated with exercise. In 1976, scientists announced the discovery of endorphins, a protein structurally similar to morphine which was later linked to the decidedly unscientific notion of runner's high.[41] But regardless of the brain chemistry involved, once you've felt the exercise state-of-mind, you want it back. You're hooked.

When most men think of exercise, they think of jogging through an early morning landscape, pumping iron in the gym, or powering a backhand past an opponent caught flat-footed across the net. Completing the picture is a hard body, animal magnetism, and great sex deep into the night.

True, sexual fitness involves more than a well-conditioned body, as the rest of this book details. But essentially the act of sex *is* physical, based as it is in the reproductive reality of sperm finding egg. And physical exercise is *the* ticket for bumping general wellness into robust fitness—being ready, willing, and able for high-level physical performance, in bed and elsewhere. As if a prize for your commitment to exercise, don't be surprised to feel new mental clarity and more emotional stability as well.

So, will exercise turn you into the astonishing love machine you've always dreamed of being? Will an extra set of bench presses in the gym or an extra twenty laps in the pool help you in bed? Is there a special workout to keep Mr. Winkie fit and responsive for years to come?

Stay tuned: we'll answer those questions and more in this chapter.

GET MOTIVATED

You're surprised by a mischievous glint in her eye. An energetic kiss. And, if you're lucky, a hand sliding up your leg. Hel-lo! You just received call for vigorous sex. No man wants to respond with weakness. Hey, strength is our traditional hallmark. We're supposed to be strong. Period. No matter that few of us build brute strength on the job anymore.

In addition to the strength of a bull, we're also supposed to have the endurance for a hard week's work, mowing the lawn, coaching a little league team, *and* prolonged thrusting in the sack. For years on end.

Well guess what, it doesn't just happen. Maybe it did in your thrilling days of yesteryear, but fitness now means getting off your duff and exercising. Regularly. The first surprise is how good exercise feels, during and afterwards. The second surprise is that the more you do it, the easier it becomes. So get serious, and get moving.

EXERCISE 101

Sexual fitness stems from overall good health, and both are enhanced by regular exercise. Generally speaking, an ideal exercise program promotes:

- *Endurance*, through aerobic exercises
- *Strength*, through strength training
- *Flexibility*, through stretching

Not surprisingly, those are also the three main components to peak sexual conditioning too. Commit to developing all three and you stand a good chance of supercharging your metabolism, confidence—and sex life. Research has shown that people who exercise tend to have more sex than their inactive counterparts.[42] And an active lifestyle may contribute to keeping sexual passion alive as you age.[43]

Each man, at every stage of life, has his individual body type and condition. Find out how fit you are and create reasonable fitness goals. Your doctor can help there, and should be consulted before starting any new exercise program.

Now let's take a closer look at how each form of exercise works its magic.

AEROBIC TRAINING: BOOST ENDURANCE, HELP YOUR HEART

Get that heart pumping and good things happen.

Only in the past few decades have we understood why sustained, moderately-intense exercise delivers major health and fitness benefits. It took the Industrial Revolution, a sedentary work force, labor-saving gadgets, and various forms of cardiovascular disease to make us see the light.

So exactly what is aerobic activity? Simply put, any activity that significantly raises your heartbeat for at least 20 minutes. When you exercise, your muscles need more oxygen, which is part of the fuel that powers them. The heart has to pump faster to deliver the oxygen in blood from lungs to muscles.

Aerobic exercise performed regularly tones the heart muscle so it works easier and more efficiently, as does exercise during other day-to-day activities like mowing the lawn or moving in rhythmic union with your lover on a blanket in the woods.

Aerobic activity pushes more blood through veins and arteries, keeping them more elastic, cleaner, and less likely to clog and cause debilitating or fatal diseases. This is important for your sex life too, since a penis depends on the free flow of blood for an erection. For the long term, there's not a much better guarantee of sexual fitness than proper eating and regular exercise.

Getting Started

Aerobic exercise is easy to start. No room-size fitness machines or intimidating postures necessary. Just pick one or more of the following activities, check with your doctor to make sure they are appropriate for you, warm up properly, and go!

Walking

It's the simplest of the heart-friendly, endurance-building, fat-burning aerobic exercises. Just get out and walk for twenty minutes, three times this

Find Your Aerobic Training Zone

So how often and how hard and how long should you exercise to get the most cardiovascular benefits? This will vary for everyone's individual condition and goals. But there are guidelines for *frequency, intensity, and duration* of aerobic exercise.

Frequency: three to five days of exercise a week is optimal, depending on individual variables.

Intensity and duration: determined by your training zone. Learn how to know when you're exercising hard enough (but not too hard) and long enough. An informal method is simply to exercise intensely enough to feel your breathing get deeper, but not so you can't talk at the same time.

A more formal method is a formula based on your heart rate. The goal is to find your aerobic range, which is approximately 70 to 85 percent of your maximum heart rate. Here's how to do it: subtract your age from 220. Multiply that result (which is your maximum heart rate) first by .70 (for 70%) or by .85 (for 85%) to get your *training zone* expressed in heart beats per minute.

Next time you're exercising, take your pulse, either on your wrist or neck, for ten seconds and multiply that by 6 (for one minute). Bingo! If it's 70% to 85% of your maximum heart rate, you're in your training zone. That's the ideal intensity for your workout.

How much exercise is enough? The goal is to spend 20-30 minutes, but generally not more than one hour, in your training zone. Keep in mind, as your condition improves, that after about twenty minutes of aerobic exercise, your muscles start to call for fat to burn. That's when aerobic exercise turns into a real fat burner.

week. Just like that you leave the silent league of wide-waisted couch potatoes, and you're on the road to lasting health and peak sexual fitness.

Once you're walking, expand your new fitness routine and compound the rewards and fun. Many aerobic activities call for the great outdoors, and the pleasure of natural surroundings help keep you motivated.

Running

If your condition and age allow, consider picking up the pace from walking to a comfortable jog. The more intense your workouts, the greater the benefits. You might start with an easy jog and work up to a more ambitious run. Be careful to gauge the impact of increased intensity. Running can be tough on knees and ankles, but for enthusiasts nothing can match the elegant simplicity or profound psychological effects of a good run. Use good quality running shoes and replace them every six months. And try a surface like sand or grass to minimize the impact of hard surfaces like asphalt.

Swimming

It's quiet. Easy on the joints. And a wonderful full-body workout unlike any other. Make this great stress-buster even better by swimming in a pond, lake, river, or ocean whenever possible. Equipment expenses are minimal (in a pool, use goggles to avoid eye irritation). And that skimpy swimsuit is a super way to show off your new muscle definition. Go ahead, enjoy it— the ladies certainly do.

Cycling

Strap on your helmet and start peddling. Whether you head down the road or up the dirt path, the aerobic benefits rate high. Even if you choose not to focus on cycling, it adds welcome variety to your training routine. You cover more territory so there's plenty of interesting stuff to look at. The speed's a thrill. And if it's strong thighs you're after, look no further. So get into the motion, whether it's zooming past oak trees and raspberry bushes, chasing taxis down 8th Avenue, or reading the sports page on a stationary bike in the gym.

And if you can, weave cycling right into your daily life. Commuting by bike is great exercise, and it sure beats sitting in your car in bumper to bumper traffic, stress building in the chest like a blast furnace. Hey, that's you on your two thin tires, face washed with air, speeding toward fitness and well-being.

Cross-Country Skiing

Most aerobic exercises are great ways to socialize, and cross-country skiing is one of the best. Now you're pumping along a glistening white trail in a snow-softened wonderland, your lover close behind (or just in front, depending on your respective conditioning), sharing much more than a workout. And you can't help visualizing the two of you collapsing into each other's arms later in front of the fireplace.

But first things first, mister. Skiing demands conditioning. Prepare for the snow-covered trails by strength training and stretching exercises focused on the legs, lower back, and abdominal muscles. And—all right already—those are her muscles to massage while getting her in the mood in front of the fireplace.

TRY INTERVAL TRAINING

Aerobic training is terrific for cardiovascular health, but limited for building strength and burning fat. So many trainers now emphasize interval training. The idea is to integrate periods of high intensity exertion into your normal pace of exercising.

Say you're running. In interval training, you'd add a few sprints to your usual pace. Why? The high intensity sprints strengthen your muscles in a way that the slower pace doesn't. When highly stressed, muscles are forced to rebuild themselves, a process which leaves them slightly stronger than before.

Also, the sprints change your muscles' fuel. When your muscles are stressed they use fat in their fuel mix instead of carbohydrates. This is called anaerobic exercise, and differs from the aerobic type which burns carbohydrates for much of the workout. Also, stressed muscles continue their rebuilding—and fat-burning—after the exercise is over, unlike aerobic exercise, which does burn fat, but only after its store of carbohydrates is gone, and only during the exercise itself.

So interval training combines aerobic training (moderate intensity, endurance-building) with anaerobic training (high-intensity, strength-building) in the same exercise.

Combining two different exercises, such as swimming and weightlifting, offers the same advantages, only more so. Hence, a new recommendation by the American College

---

Pick a Reason...

Exercise enhances sexual fitness directly—and also promotes good sex by helping to: boost immunity, keep weight in check, reduce risk of heart disease, prevent prostate cancer, defuse stress, boost vitality, increase strength, raise HDL (good cholesterol) and lower LDL (bad cholesterol), eliminate constipation, soothe anxiety, stop tension headaches, enjoy better sleep, boost mood, prevent type II diabetes, boost self-esteem—and more![44]

of Sports Medicine for at least two sessions of strength-training a week in addition to regular aerobic exercise.[45]

In-Line Skating

Call it poetry in motion. Aerobic flow. Or any other lyrical phrase that captures the graceful fluidity of in-line skating. Of course, the poetry ends abruptly when you fall. But if you've equipped yourself with a good helmet and proper pads and guards, you simply get up, dust yourself off, and get back in the groove. When starting, avoid too much ground time by enrolling in an instructional clinic at the local sports shop. One of the first things taught is how to fall properly, which for a beginner is the most helpful tip of all. Your confidence rockets when you learn the basics well.

As in some other aerobic activities, your legs get a fantastic workout while skating, but your upper body doesn't. So combine skating with weight training on alternate days to balance endurance with strength. And of course, warm up and stretch often to stay supple and able to get into...well, the poetry of it.

Kayaking, Canoeing, Rowing

Think of it as boating with all-natural engines—your arms. These classic rides tone your heart and lungs while adding arm and chest strength. And who can say exactly what benefits come from intimate contact with ocean, lake, or river? Maybe some day we'll know. In the meantime, greet a loon or pelican for a social change of pace.

The big time upper-body workouts with paddles or oars combine wonderfully with cycling or running on land-locked days.

Aerobic Classes

Classes offer precision aerobic exercise and music and people in controlled exhilaration. Sure, the ladies probably outnumber men, but you can handle that, right? Scheduled classes also help you nourish your commitment to exercise. When a gym is on or near your commuting route, classes are a stress-busting, reinvigorating transition from workplace to home. Instructors help you choose the aerobic class that's perfect for you, from dance to step to low-intensity. And since you're there, it's an easy walk over to the free weights or machines for strength-training.

Avoid Overtraining

The father of aerobics—the man who introduced the word in 1976— now warns about the dangers of training too zealously. In *Dr. Kenneth Cooper's Antioxidant Revolution*, he states that stressing the muscles beyond their capacity creates free radicals which can lead to a host of degenerative diseases, such as cancer and cardiovascular ills.[46]

Free radicals are unstable oxygen molecules that attract and damage nearby molecules, and start chain reactions leading toward disease. The antioxidants mentioned in his title refer to nutritional elements which protect cells from free radicals. Taking Vitamins E and C, selenium, and a daily dose of beta carotene are considered good basic supplementation.

How much exercise is too much? When you exhaust yourself with many high-intensity workouts and feel constantly tired, it's time to reconsider your routine.

Sports

Times are changing, guy. Remember when school gym classes were feasts of competition—kickball, baseball, football, etc.? Nowadays, fitness training is moving in strong. Which makes sense when you look at the alarming statistics of overweight adolescents. Turns out that baseball, while rating high in the national consciousness as true sport, rates low as an aerobic activity.

Nonetheless, for many of us, sports are here to stay. It's just wise to rate your favorites and gauge their contribution to your cardiovascular health. When you look at sports in that light, you see a range of aerobic benefits. Soccer, for instance, rates high on the endurance-building scale, with golf low. If you need convincing, play a few minutes of flat-out soccer, and note how your legs and lungs feel (if you're not breathing too hard to think straight). Sure, it's good to get out and walk on those emerald fairways, and uniquely satisfying (especially following those classic shots when you've hammered the sweet spot and watched the ball flying long and straight far down the middle of the fairway). Just don't think of it as intense aerobics.

Aerobically, basketball gets the nod. Progressively lower on the cardiovascular scale lie tennis, volleyball, bowling, and fishing. But hey, you're trolling along that weedy shoreline trying to outsmart a crafty largemouth bass, not exercise your heart. So why not take a good constitutional after cleaning the campfire frying pan?

Sex

And you thought baseball was satisfying! Ah, sex. What a great workout. Unless you're into convoluted Kama Sutra postures, which demand serious strength and flexibility, endurance is the key here. Of course being strong and supple help, and so does that new muscle definition your exercise routine has created.

All your fitness training gives you a leg up in the sex department. Your heart's strong and able to power thrusts of whatever intensity and duration. Your blood vessels are elastic and unobstructed, delivering a high volume of plasmic erection fluid on demand. And your head's clear. Man, it doesn't get any better than this. Especially when emotional intimacy compliments your physical fitness, enfolding the whole enterprise with passion and fulfillment.

STRENGTH TRAINING: BUILD MUSCLE, BURN FAT

Years ago, the classic Charles Atlas ad offered a simple choice for the beach: be the muscular guy kicking sand or the weakling getting showered by it. Needless to say, the weakling wasn't the one with the girl.

Fortunately, we've moved beyond that image (except for the occasional muscle-bound meathead). Today there are many good reasons for integrating strength training into your life—and many ways to do so. Better sex is only one reason, though for sure a very good one.

Strength training is still a story about muscles, because increased strength comes from increased muscle mass. Let's take a look at the whys and hows of beefing up.

Five Great Reasons To Strength-Train

- *Build self-esteem.* True, most of us aren't focused on sculpted bodies slathered in oil and flexing on-stage in a body building contest. But most men—and women—naturally prefer some muscular definition over the bean-pole look. And that goes double for the naked body. Muscles are certainly not all there is to sexual confidence, but they sure help.

- *Boost capability* in athletics, moving furniture, opening jars— and sex. There is something called athletic sex and muscles are part of it. A big part. As we've seen, strength training is for strength; aerobics is for endurance. But the same distinction also exists *within* strength training—you can focus on muscular strength or muscular endurance.

Again, it depends on your body type and why you're training. And your sexual preferences.

If you enjoy more athletic sex (such as standing and supporting your lover as she straddles you during intercourse), obviously you'll need more muscular strength. However, in sitting intercourse, while strength still plays a part, muscular endurance comes more into play.

- *Burn fat.* As your metabolism rises, so does your ability to burn fat. Muscles can burn fat as fuel—so the more muscle, the more fat-burning activity. Weight loss becomes less important as your body composition shifts in the direction of less fat and more muscle (muscle weighs more than fat). Dieting becomes less important because you don't necessarily have to eat less to lose weight. Think of it in terms of body mechanics. Building your muscles helps to create that sex machine called a well-conditioned male who can do more, longer, in and out of bed.

- *Keep bones aligned, healthy, and pain-free.* The skeletal and muscular systems work together smoothly—when everything functions in harmony. But injured or weakened muscles can wreak havoc with the natural alignment of bones and joints. Strong and supple muscles are good insurance against the aches and pains that put one on the reserve list. And there's nothing sexy about being on the reserve list!

- *Complement aerobics.* Cross training develops optimum strength, endurance, and flexibility. An alternate-day schedule of strength training and aerobics, for instance, builds your capacities while allowing specific muscles the rest they require for optimum growth and maintenance.

Start By Building Motivation

Strength training—that's pumping iron, right? Barbells and bench presses and bulging biceps? Well, yes. But you can also build strength using the fitness machines that have become so popular at gyms and fitness centers, and by doing old-fashioned calisthenics like pushups and sit-ups.

There are good reasons to use all of the above. Keeping your interest level up is one. Ray Kybartas, a top trainer in California and author of *Fitness is Religion*, stresses the benefits of constantly evolving your exercise routines.[47] Variation keeps you from getting bored, so you keep exercising and getting stronger and more fit.

How Muscles Grow

You build a muscle by stressing and then resting it. That process lies at the heart of strength training. When you work a muscle intensely, on a microscopic level you destabilize its tissues.[48] The muscle responds by rebuilding itself. And when you really stress the muscle, say by lifting weights in repetitions you can barely complete, the muscle rebuilds itself slightly larger and stronger than it was before. Hey presto: bigger muscles.

Sufficient rest after high-intensity contractions allows the muscle enough time to properly rebuild itself. So it's important to rest between sets in weight lifting, and to wait at least 48 hours between workouts, or to work different muscles on successive days.

So should a beginner hit the gym and lift weights that make his eyeballs bulge? Obviously not. All strength training isn't high-intensity lifting. Every individual should target specific goals along the continuum between strength and endurance training, and start toward reasonable goals slowly.

The best way to get motivated and stay that way is to learn how to train properly. And the best way to do that is by learning from a qualified trainer. But there are also many books and videos available to help. The important thing is to get out there and get started. Whether you use free weights or machines is less important than whether you're using them regularly to build and maintain muscle mass.

Seven Tips For Successful Strength Training

1. *Warm up and Stretch*

   Warming up and stretching are not interchangeable. Warm up before you stretch. Just a few minutes jogging in place or up and down stairs will do. Then stretch to get muscles prepared to work out. Don't overdo it and don't bounce muscles in a stretch. Listen to your body.

2. *Set Goals*

   As with just about every other activity, knowing what you want to accomplish helps define how you'll get there. Are you interested primarily in strength, size, or toning? If you're new to these considerations, a personal trainer is invaluable. It might sound like a luxury, but all it takes is two or three sessions to learn the basics. And he or she will teach you the proper use of weights, which is essential to avoid strains or injury, especially if you're using free weights.

3. *Develop a Core Routine*

   Start with major muscle groups, as in thighs, lower legs, back, chest, arms, and abdominals. You don't have to become an exercise physiologist but you should know what muscles you're working in any given exercise. In the thighs, for instance, one exercise works the quadriceps in front and another works the hamstrings in back. Once you've got the major muscles covered, you can refine your workout keeping your goals in mind.

4. *Build Up your Workout Gradually*

   Generally, you should be shooting for eight to ten repetitions in two sets for each lift. The weight should be sufficient to make more than that difficult or impossible. Build up to more weight incrementally.

5. *Never Jerk Weights Up or Down.*

   Lift with a smooth, steady motion. That promotes muscle strength while minimizing injury to joints.

6. *Lift at Least Twice a Week But No More Than Every Other Day*

   Remember that your muscles need a chance to rebuild after being stressed. Lifting too often interferes with that process. When you have your routine organized into major muscle groups, you can split it up and work out on successive days, as long as each group gets the necessary rest. That's a good way to reduce the time any given session takes.

7. *Do Your Strength Sexercises*

   You don't need a gym to exercise the most important set of muscles directly relating to sexuality. Your pelvic floor muscles influence how and when you ejaculate, and can help keep your prostate gland healthy too. Specific workouts for those muscles are called Kegel exercises, which are important enough to warrant their own chapter. If you haven't already read it, don't miss it.

FLEXIBILITY TRAINING: BE SUPPLE, MOVE FREELY

Flexibility is too often undervalued. Regularly stretching muscles, tendons, and ligaments prepares you for wide-ranging free movement and pain-free performance in bed and elsewhere.

With a supple body, you're not only more likely to avoid aches, pains, and injury that put you out of service, you're also ready for advanced sexual positions literally out of reach for your stiff and out-of-shape peers.

Warm Up—*then* Stretch

Yes, you should warm up before stretching just as seriously as you'd warm up for running or lifting. It doesn't take much, just some easy walking or a slow and simple version of whatever exercise might follow. Slow, circular rotations of as many joints as you have time for helps too. There are good reasons for doing so. Warmed, elastic muscles are much less prone to strain or injury, and ready for peak action sooner. Also, a full body warm-up reduces the chances of one muscle remaining tight and causing a related muscle to strain in compensation. So warm up first!

Some men think of stretching as "warming up." While the two certainly overlap, warming up is merely a prelude to some other activity. Stretching can be an end in itself, the third indispensable link in the Fit-For-Sex physical fitness triad.

Establish a rhyme and reason for stretching. Stretch specific muscles and muscle systems. This can be done in many ways: from first thing in the morning by yourself, to sensuous, shared stretching which transforms naturally into foreplay at night.

Stretching promotes general health and fitness, and the free movement in muscles directly involved in sex.

Five Great Reasons To Stretch

1. *Increase Suppleness and Flexibility*

   Men often develop strength at the expense of flexibility. The advantages of strength are offset when movement is restricted by tight or stiff muscles. Anyway, sex is much more about fluid movement (as well as the movement of fluids) than brute strength. By boosting the lubrication of joints, tendons, and ligaments, stretching encourages suppleness and grace. In short, stretching can make you better prepared for the range of movements in sex.

2. *Boost Sensitivity*

   The slow, quiet nature of stretching encourages awareness of your body. You can—and should—listen to the subtle cues in muscles and joints as you stretch. Find and respect your limits; they come from your body, not from a rule book. The inner quiet which enhances physical awareness also encourages emotional and mental openness, as well as the intimacy defining a mature sexual relationship.

3. *Calm Your Mind and Nerves*

   Great sex requires presence. Stretching relaxes your body and mind, leaving you more open to the pleasures of sex.

4. *Build Vitality*

   Fatigue is often the result of low levels of activity and a restricted range of movement. A good stretching routine increases circulation and encourages deep breathing, both of which can provide an energy boost.

5. *Avoid Strain and Injury*

   When you warm-up and stretch regularly, you keep muscles in balance. Too often we tend to favor one group of muscles which naturally work in opposition to another. That imbalance can cause overcompensation by the stronger ones, causing misalignment of bones and joints. The result can be stiffness, pain, or injury. Stretching helps keep the muscular and skeletal systems properly aligned, in balance, and fit for the fullness of movement in sex.

   > **Flexibility Gauge**
   >
   > How do you know when you need to stretch before sex? Sore muscles afterward tell you so. Everything from dull aches to searing back pain can be your body's way of saying you were too cold or tight for sex.

Five Stretches for Sexual Fitness

Now that we know why to stretch, here are the basics of how. Remember, begin slowly. Don't bounce or strain. A good basic routine stretches large muscle groups first: back, sides, pelvis, groin, calves, and thighs. We'll concentrate on stretching for overall sexual fitness. Breathe deeply and easily throughout. And of course, warm up first. Here are five basic stretches for sexual fitness. Explore others with a personal trainer or yoga instructor.

1. *Lower Back*

   Get on your hands and knees, with your back straight. Now arch your back as far up as you comfortably can and hold for a few seconds. Then lower your belly, dropping your back to the opposite position. Repeat. When you raise your back, tilt your pelvis forward as if thrusting during intercourse. Conversely, when lowering your back, tilt your pelvis back as if withdrawing during intercourse. Remember, there's

nothing sensual about back pain. Keeping your back flexible is the key
to back health and the foundation of good sex.

2. *Upper Back and Sides*

   Stand with your feet together, back straight, and arms at your sides.
   Slowly raise your arms until they are parallel with the floor. Relax and
   drop your shoulders. Now continue raising your arms until they are
   directly above your shoulders. Keep your back straight. Stretch up for
   a few seconds. Hold. Then relax and slowly drop your arms.

   Repeat, this time putting your palms together above your head. Then
   slowly bend to the left, keeping your arms straight. Hold. Bend back
   straight and slightly to the other side. Hold. Bend back up straight and
   slowly lower your arms back down to your sides.

3. *Groin*

   Sit with a straight back and your feet drawn up to your body, soles of
   your feet touching each other. Now lower your knees out to the side.
   Again, only to the point of a gentle stretch. Don't overextend. Hold and
   release. Repeat.

4. *Hips*

   Lie on your back with your legs extended and resting on the floor. Pull
   one leg up and with hands behind the thigh, gently stretch it toward
   your chest. Hold. Repeat with the other leg.

5. *Thighs*

   Stand facing with your front to a wall and lean on it with your left
   hand slightly for support. Lift your right foot up behind you and grab
   it with your right hand, gently pulling it in to your buttocks. Hold and
   release. Repeat with your other leg. This stretches the quadriceps muscles in the front of your thighs.

   For the hamstrings in the back of your thighs, sit on a bed or bench
   and extend your right leg on its surface, its knee straight, with your left
   leg on the floor. Gently bend from your waist toward your right toes.
   Try to keep your spine straight and don't push too far. Hold. Repeat
   with the other leg.

   Forget that no-pain-no-gain stuff. Pain has no place in stretching. The
   idea here is to gently stretch your muscles and joints, relax your mind
   and body, and get into some great sex.

FANTASY

You're eating a late dinner in a dark restaurant. An attractive dark-haired woman in a simple black dress with curves in all the right places asks to join you. Sure, you say, be my guest. She sits surprisingly close and the two of you make small talk and laugh for a few minutes. Then she puts her hand on your thigh and gently squeezes it. You do the same and find her warm and responsive to your touch, so you move your hand under her dress and slide it up her smooth thigh and feel a garter belt but no underwear. She leans over and kisses you with her full lips while spreading her legs and moving your hand onto her moist...

Greetings from the realm of fantasy, where every woman is beautiful, hot, and willing. No commitments or deadlines ever cramp your style, which ranges from firmly assertive to scandalously wild. You can return often and leave in an instant. It's beautiful, baby.

Or is it? If fantasies are so swell, why do we tend to feel guilty about them, and rarely share them with anyone except lovers, if then?

GOOD NEWS FROM FANTASYLAND

Bob Berkowitz, author of *Male Sexual Fantasies*, reports that the "Testosterone Curtain" is falling; that men are finally beginning to open up about their fantasies, just like women did to their benefit twenty years ago.[49] If true, it's a welcome shift as men move beyond their classic one-dimensional silence to a willingness to share the details on the erotic cinema screens of their imaginations.

Sexual fantasies can play a positive role in psychological sexual fitness. They can boost our arousal, provide a healthy escape from pressure-filled lives, feed our confidence, and soothe our anxieties. In other words, they can provide simple pleasures and support, and safe sexual rehearsals.

However, if fantasizing begins to interfere with reality, becoming obsessive in nature or accompanied by strong urges to act out fantasies to the detriment of oneself or others, that's a different story, and could signal the need for psychological counseling. But what most of us inwardly envision day in and day out is no more than a healthy expression of our wide-ranging inner lives.

Carl Jung, the Swiss psychiatrist we'll meet again in *Midlife*, said fantasies originate from the same source as the dreams we have while asleep at night, but experience while awake, as day-dreams.[50] As such, fantasies arise from our unconscious, which underlies our thinking minds and, according to Jung, connects us with the ground of our being, and our highest potential.

But what's also interesting about his view is that fantasies present us with thoughts and feelings which are "compensatory to the situation or attitude of the conscious mind."[51] This is a very helpful tool for learning from, and not just observing, our daydreams and fantasies. More about this in a moment.

But before considering what sexual fantasies might mean for us, let's first explore what they are.

ENJOY A SAFE HAVEN

Sexual fantasies—erotic daydreams and images—occur anytime and anywhere, before or during sex or while mowing the lawn or driving to work. We can actively create fantasies or they can happen on their own. Some men fantasize many times a day, while others do so less frequently or not at all. Both men and women have sexual fantasies, although generally not of the same type.

The classic difference is that men are more likely to visualize female bodies and/or to be the active partner in sex with strangers, whereas women's sexual fantasies include love and relationships, as evidenced by 200 million romance novels sold every year by one publishing company alone.[52] Of course, those are just two ends of the spectrum. Men's fantasies can include intimate scenarios involving present or former lovers, whereas many women daydream about anonymous sex or even rape, which is one good example of fantasies that aren't about sex the fantasizer wants in reality, but simply within the safety of the imagination.

Of course, that's just the beginning. Here's a sampling of the kinds of fantasies men commonly experience.

Anonymous Sex

"She's standing near me at the bus station and smiles seductively when I approach her and ask for directions. I've got a car outside, I say, why don't we take a ride..."

Fantasies of anonymous sex are commonplace. And that's no surprise, since they offer an uncomplicated and successful version of real-world sex—without concerns of safe sex, etiquette, or her preferences. In the real world, such concerns broaden a man and his sense of fulfillment. Not so with fantasy, a world without arguments, commitments, or schedules. It's about pure pleasure, providing a relaxing interlude for the modern male juggling this role, that duty, day in and day out. Hey, it's fast and easy. Is that a bad thing?

Anonymity extends to fantasies involving prostitutes. For men who would never consider buying sex in reality, doing so in fantasy is safe, certainly no strain on the wallet, and even saves a drive to the seedy side of town.

Group Sex

"The blond was lying on her back with her legs spread, moaning with pleasure as her brunette friend satisfied her with her tongue. I watched and waited patiently, my sap rising, ready to take the tag and move in next..."

Groups start with three and the ménage à trois is a highly popular starting point. Here the fantasist isn't involved with the messy emotions that simultaneous relationships inevitably bring. And he compounds the pleasures of even the most singular fantasy with one woman. Again, while watching or interacting with one or both women, a man doesn't have to bear responsibility for real world emotions—he's too busy! And watching two women is a big turn-on too, as proven by its prevalence in pornographic images.

Speaking of which, how does pornography relate to fantasy? Well, they're intimately entwined. But here we're simply separating them into images on the inside (fantasy) and those supplied from outside. More on the latter in *Pornography*.

Homosexual Sex

"I was lying on the beach with my eyes closed. A shadow crossed my face and I looked up into the eyes of a classic hunk standing over me wearing nothing but cut off jeans, with the sun turning his blond hair into a golden mane..."

In a society with a deep chasm between homosexual and heterosexual values, having a pleasurable fantasy about such a threatening subject can be very troubling for a heterosexual man. Yet June Reinisch, author of *The Kinsey Institute New Report on Sex*, cites one report that says homosexual fantasies are among the most frequently occurring for straight men.[53] Chances are it's just that restless, unconscious male mind wondering what this cordoned-off area holds. But again, when this or any fantasy begins to trouble you with its persistence, or interferes with your real social or work life, talking with someone about it can help, especially a psychologist trained to help you understand your thoughts and feelings.

Public Sex

"We leaned against the rail at the scenic overlook to watch the sunset. The silence was broken only by an occasional car passing on the highway, and the few people around us had started heading back to their cars. We looked at each other and smiled, hugged and kissed, and I slowly lifted her T-shirt over her head, her shorts down her soft legs, and moved behind her..."

Why not do it in public—privately? It's the freedom, the simple turn-on, and clear benefit of sexual fantasy—doing the wild thing in the open without being carted away in a paddy wagon.

Fringe Sex

"Answering a personal ad for a "SWM," I realized the "W" should have been an "&". She opened her door wearing a black silk robe, walked into the living room while shedding it, and stood waiting for me wearing nothing but a black leather corset and holding a black silk scarf..."

Whoa! If you're not ready for this, many other men are, at least in fantasy. Whether or not they admit it, they're interested in being bound, and/or binding someone else. This is the Sadomasochism (S&M) spectrum within the larger spectrum of sexual fantasy. Here's a gentle spanking, there's some sort of strange table; here's a willing sex slave, there's an ominous surgical device. At this point, caution flags come up. This is dangerous territory, which of course is exactly its appeal. But the familiar rule applies: if the fantasy doesn't intrude into your real life, with dangerous ramifications, fine. But if you begin to need the fantasy to satisfy yourself sexually, or when you're strongly tempted to act it out, putting yourself or anyone else at risk—stop! Think twice. Seek help.

SIX TIPS FOR FANTASIZING

More men are beginning to be comfortable accepting their sexual fantasies—and sharing them, which can be as important as simply being turned on by them. Here's a short list of guidelines for living with fantasies.

1. *Enjoy Them*

   When a fantasy turns you on and causes no one problems, just enjoy it! If it feels good, do it! Don't worry if you see yourself in women's underwear, or find yourself having sex with an animal! It's not real, it's easy and safe.

2. *Share Them*

   Of course enjoying your fantasies solo is fine. But relationships can pass a milestone when partners share their sexual fantasies. Nancy Friday, in her groundbreaking book on women's fantasies tells her own story of what she thought was a close boyfriend getting out of bed and leaving when she revealed one of her fantasies.[54] Times are changing, and thank goodness for that. Yes, some fantasies can be shocking and the appropriateness of sharing each fantasy has to be judged individually within each relationship. But when lovers share fantasies they can add spice to sex as well as deepen knowledge of each other's preferences.

3. *Act Them Out*

   Role-playing turns many couples on. Sure, you won't want to broadcast your favorite scenes at the coffee machine, but in the privacy of your bedroom, this is the safe way to bring your fantasies, and their excitement, to life. Of course this means fantasies that don't hurt anyone. Dressing up, or down, are two examples. Try supercharging the seduction on "French night," add a touch of intrigue on bondage night— whatever works, doesn't threaten anyone, and turns you both on.

4. *Shape Them*

   Maurice Yaffé, sex therapist and author of *Sexual Happiness for Men*, suggests "shaping" fantasies while masturbating to alter sexual preferences that might be causing problems in a relationship.[55] He proposes that a man use whatever offending fantasy to turn himself on, if necessary, and then actively guide the fantasy into safer sexual territory and satisfy himself there. He also notes that when fantasies can't be changed and are causing major problems, medications are available to eliminate them. Obviously, psychotherapy is appropriate in these conditions. Also, powerful ideas about alternatives to fantasies are found in *Tantric Sex*.

5. *Learn From Them*

   So what does a fantasy mean? That depends on each fantasy, each person, and each culture that person lives in. Just as every culture has different ideas and values about sex, so does every person. Fantasies are not beamed from an exterior source (that's pornography). They arise from within. As mentioned above, some psychologists say fantasies reveal something about ourselves, possibly compensating for conscious attitudes or actions that are leading us away from our true desire or true needs. For instance, if we dream of being forced into sex with a dominating woman, perhaps we need to let go of some controlling aspect of our lives. But to explore such individual examples, working with a qualified therapist is optimal.

6. *Affirm With Them*

Affirmations are spreading. From gymnasts to bobsledders, athletes have discovered the power of succeeding by visualizing success. It's the power of positive thinking. Say "I can," and improve the chances that you will. Consider applying this to sex. A fantasy can be a rehearsal. Practice, in effect. And as such it can build your self-confidence. This is not suggesting fantasy as a substitute for intimacy, or stressing technique above connection. But visualizing sex can help you explore whatever aspect of it that currently attracts you. It's the positive road to success.

FERTILITY

In the dim recesses of human prehistory, sex and pregnancy were unrelated phenomena. No one connected a romp in the cave to L'il Neanderthal's appearance nine months later. Then while civilizing ourselves we gradually realized the profound consequences of the act.

In recent decades, our understanding of conception has skyrocketed, along with our ability to help couples conceive—good news given research that shows a decline in male and female fertility. How are guys faring in the fertility department? Depends on who you ask. In terms of sperm count, the experts are divided. Some say there has been no drop overall. Others cite statistics which show male sperm count dropping almost by half between 1940 and 1990, with the average *quantity* of sperm declining by nearly 20%.[56] Alarming if true.

But for some men, statistics are much less important than discovering how their partners can have a successful pregnancy. If you're among them, here's important news and information about fertility.

THE EYE-POPPING BIOLOGY OF MULTIPLICATION[57]

In one ejaculation, a man can release up to 400 million sperm. 40-50 million per milliliter of ejaculate (figure 2 to 3 milliliters per average ejaculate) is considered normal, however; below that currently qualifies as low sperm count. But as we'll see, quantity is not the only factor of sperm's effectiveness; it has to be able to move well too.

Each sperm contains 23 chromosomes, half the genetic blueprint required to make a human being. Like *serious* Fedex guys, a sperm's sole mission is to deliver that genetic package or die trying. Only one will successfully accomplish its mission.

Sperm are created in the testes, the male sex glands or gonads that hang in the sack-like scrotum (and yes, it's natural for one to hang lower than the other). The testes are round-the-clock sperm factories which crank out massive amounts of sperm every day. They're working hard even as you read these words. The sperm are produced in tiny, coiled tubes called seminiferous tubules; they pass through the tubules and are stored outside the testes in another tube called the epididymis (the testes plus the epididymis make up the testicles).

By the time a sperm cell reaches the epididymis, it may have swum more than the length of two football fields in internal plumbing. But the most remarkable part of its journey is yet to come. When a man is sufficiently sexually stimulated, the epididymis begins to pulsate, forcing the sperm through another tube called the vas deferens, and then into the urethra, the tube that leads to the outside world. At the same time, the sperm is surrounded by nourishing and protective fluids secreted by a series of glands: the seminal vesicles, the prostate gland and the Cowper's glands. The sperm and the soup it swims in can now be called semen. Thanks to that wonder of nature we call ejaculation, the plucky sperm are boldly sent where they've never been before: the female vagina.

Meanwhile...

The male reproductive system is geared towards quantity: delivering so many sperm improves the odds that at least one will hit the jackpot. The woman, however, has the pleasure of hosting this little party. And while men are creating millions of sperm a day, she's carefully preparing just one of their counterpart—the egg—every month.

Every woman is born with as many eggs as she'll ever have. Which is plenty more than she'll ever use, since each of her two ovaries contains about 400,000 of them. Once every 28 days or so, beginning at puberty, one egg develops and moves to the wall of the ovary and is ejected—a process called ovulation.

Like a sperm, the egg has some traveling to do to reach its destiny. After ovulation, the egg is drawn into the funnel-shaped opening of the fallopian tube, where fertilization occurs. The fertilized egg then travels into the uterus.

Let's get back to our heroes. When we last left the sperm, a few hundred million of the little guys had just been blasted out of the only home they ever knew into the new environs of the vagina. About half or more of them end up swimming the wrong way, out of the vagina, never to be heard from again. Others get tired and simply stop wriggling. But millions do reach the fallopian tubes, after swimming for anywhere from an hour to a couple of days, where many will make a wrong turn and enter the fallopian tube without the egg. More will just conk out before they get to the finish line. At this point it becomes obvious why so many are called to do the job.

If there is a waiting egg, by the time the sperm in the right fallopian tube reaches it, numbers will have dwindled to a matter of dozens. They swarm around the egg, which is many times larger than they are, each trying to be the first to penetrate its protective coating with a dissolving enzyme. Just one will succeed, and its packet of chromosomes will join with the egg's to form a complete set. About 30 hours after fertilization, the egg, or zygote as it's now called, will divide, the first of many divisions that results in all the complicated structures of the human body.

GO FOR IT!

To maximize the chances for pregnancy, plan intercourse around your partner's maximum time of fertility, which is the 24-hour period in which the egg is properly positioned in her fallopian tube and ready for penetration— usually in the middle of her menstrual cycle. Because the time of ovulation varies from woman to woman and month to month, the best approach is to have sex every other day (to maximize sperm build-up) for a few days on either side of day 14 of her monthly cycle.[58]

Some doctors think that the position in which you have sex can improve the odds of conception, mainly by depositing the sperm closer to the fallopian tubes. A rear-entry position (either kneeling or lying side-by-side) fits that bill. You can minimize the amount of sperm spilling out of the vagina by removing your penis immediately after ejaculation, and by your partner lying on her back with her hips elevated on a pillow for a few minutes.[59]

SAVE THE SPERM

Sure, you've probably got millions and millions of them. But if you expect to reproduce, it won't hurt to conserve. Follow these tips to keep your swim team in top shape:

- *Cut back on the booze:* alcohol consumption can temporarily lower sperm count.
- *Skip the smoke:* both nicotine and marijuana use have also been shown to lower the quantity of healthy sperm.
- *Stay out of hot tubs:* too much heat decreases sperm production. Long hot baths, saunas, and steam rooms are included.
- *Loosen up:* some experts think tight underwear or pants heat up the testes enough to interfere with sperm production.
- *Relax:* stress can lower sperm count too. See the *Stress* chapter for tension-busting strategies. Exercise is great, but don't overdo it.

WHEN TO SEEK HELP

You've been trying. And trying. But no baby. Is there a problem?

In fact, there may not be. Only 20% of couples who try to conceive a child are successful the first time they try. One study of more than 5,000 couples found that 42% took four months or more.[60] Most experts advise that there's no reason to suspect a fertility problem until a couple's been trying to conceive for a year. But you may want to see a doctor sooner if:

- She is over age 30.
- She has a history of pelvic disease.
- She experiences painful periods, miscarriage or irregular menstrual cycles.
- You know you have a low sperm count.
- You've had mumps, or a sexually transmitted disease.
- You've injured your testicles.
- If there are other reasons to suspect a fertility problem (for example, if either of you had problems conceiving in a previous relationship).

FINDING HELP

Is it her or you who's having a problem? The likelihood is about the same: about 35% of infertility cases turn out to be a female problem, and 35% turn out to be a male problem. The remaining cases are either both, or unexplained causes. So you can see why it's important for both of you to get checked. But where do you start?

If you need a referral to a fertility clinic or specialist, two organizations that can help are: The American Society For Reproductive Medicine (205-978-5000, or http://www.asrm.org), and Resolve (617-623-0744, or www.resolve.org). Ask for their list of recommended practitioners. Then call the fertility clinics you chose and ask:

- Do they have, or work with, specialists such as a reproductive endocrinologist, gynecologist, urologist and reproductive biologist? Depending on procedures options, you might also ask about a reproductive immunologist, embryologist, reproductive urologist, and geneticist.
- What kinds of fertility problems were recently treated? Compare success rates.

- How long will their testing take? If you want to go slowly, will they accommodate you?
- What will the first visit consist of, and at what cost?

Three fertility clinics recognized as among the country's best are:

- Boston University Medical Center—Boston, MA—(617) 638-6767
- New York Hospital-Cornell Medical Center—New York, NY—(800) 822-2694
- St. Luke's Hospital—St. Louis, MO—(314) 567-1400

WHAT TO EXPECT

Fertility doctors have a whole battery of techniques they can use to figure out what is, and isn't, going on. Some of the essential tests include:[61]

- Female hormone blood test.
- Post-intercourse check.
- Fallopian tubes x-ray.
- Uterine lining biopsy.
- Out-patient surgery to check for endometriosis, and pelvic condition.
- Semen analysis.

Most male fertility problems can be grouped into four categories:

- Problems with sperm-regulating endocrine systems.
- Testes unable to produce sperm.
- Obstructions interfering with sperm storage or delivery.
- Sexual disorders (ED, etc.) which prevent sperm from being deposited in the woman.

TREATING MALE INFERTILITY

If you and your partner are having difficulty becoming pregnant, don't panic. A recent study reported in *The New England Journal of Medicine* showed the chances for getting pregnant were about equal for those seeking treatment within six months and those who postponed treatment for 12 months while continuing regular intercourse.[62] Further, the risks of treatment to conceive sooner can include multiple pregnancies as well as emotional and financial stress. So a factor to consider is how long you're willing to wait; it's often a matter not of whether you can conceive, but when. That said, there are effective male options for helping a couple conceive, such as:

- *Treating sexual disorders.* Details in the *Impotence* chapter.
- *Drug therapy* can increase sperm production by correcting hormonal imbalances. Antibiotics may also be used to treat infections that affect fertility.
- *Surgery* can remove obstructions that block sperm production or ejaculation (a vasectomy can technically be restored surgically, but the procedure is not always successful).
- *Artificial insemination* takes healthy sperm from the man, concentrates the more active sperm, and inserts them into the woman. The latest techniques can succeed with sperm acquired even from men with very low sperm count. Alternatively, sperm from a donor can be substituted.
- *In vitro fertilization* and similar procedures combine eggs and sperm in a lab. The fertilized egg is then placed in the woman, where it can develop normally.

FOREPLAY

When it comes to foreplay, guys get a bad rap. Women, the stereotype goes, like a lot of foreplay in lovemaking, while men would rather fast forward to the climax. But in fact, men's attitudes towards foreplay are varied. According to the Hite report on male sexuality, a survey of over 7,000 men, 24% of those surveyed like foreplay to last a half hour or more. Ten percent said "the longer, the better," and fortunately only 1% preferred no foreplay at all.[63]

Maybe you think of foreplay as a kind of appetizer—tasty, but not really the reason you sat down to eat. If so, you're missing out on a smorgasbord of sexual goodies. Remember, the reason every great meal is prefaced by an appetizer is not for you to wolf it down in a single bite. Rather, its purpose is to start the meal gradually, with tidbits of pleasure, and enhance the whole experience with anticipation of pleasures yet to come.

START THE BALL ROLLING

Men too often think of foreplay as kissing and touching before intercourse. But the best foreplay adds everything from soft words to a soapy massage in the bathtub, wandering fingers in the movies to oral sex. Foreplay can start early in the day—or even the day before—with whispered endearments, delivered flowers, or provocative messages on voice mail. In fact, when passion is running high, or in advanced non-ejaculation practices, foreplay can be a familiar state of being, continuously fed by casual touches, stolen kisses, and high-quality afterplay. If you're in this state now, give praise to the gods and don't change anything.

Far from being just a token nod to her enjoyment, foreplay should be cultivated like an art form because it:

- *Stimulates your bodies* to prepare for orgasm by triggering a host of physical responses, including increased nervous system impulses and blood flow to the genitals. This results in an erection for you and vaginal lubrication for her. And as many couples discover, the better the foreplay, the better the intimacy and orgasm.
- *Expresses the love* and desire you feel for your partner, without focusing on your drive to orgasm. Result: major bonus points for you in her

ongoing feminine emotional tally—points you'll draw on next time you're in the doghouse.

- *Supercharges intercourse* by giving your body time to become completely aroused. Sure, sometimes you're ready at the drop of a hat, but let's face it, not always. Then you'll appreciate foreplay's role in fanning smoldering desire into flaming arousal.

- *Equalizes your levels of arousal.* Since it generally takes longer for women to become fully aroused than men, foreplay helps insure that sex will be optimal for both. Rolling off her after a grand-slam orgasm only to notice she hasn't left first base yet will score only negative points. Make a habit of that and the only action you'll see will be solo batting practice.

FOREPLAY WITH ALL FIVE SENSES

Good foreplay includes physical and emotional stimulation, as well as trust, communication, gentleness, and enough time.

These elements are expressed in infinite variations. Every couple will find its own preferences, and discovering them can be one of the most exciting aspects of a sexual relationship. One approach to great foreplay is to involve as many of the senses as possible. Of course no rules apply. Whether you like to concentrate on just a few techniques that rock your socks, or continually sample a long list of pleasures, it's up to you—and her.

Excite with Sights

Some say that foreplay begins with a look, whether coy glances or a blatantly lustful stare. In any case, most of us respond very well to visual cues. Here are some ways to get her visually involved.

- *Set the mood.* It's hard to get in the mood when you're surrounded by ripe piles of dirty laundry, so clean up ahead of time. Turn the overhead lights off, turn on the accent lighting or light some candles. Get rid of anything distracting or unpleasant (including the pictures of your last girlfriend). If you've been living together for awhile, try getting away. A bed and breakfast in the hills, or even the motel across town, can introduce a fresh atmosphere for remaking love.

- *Look your best.* Remember way back when you first started dating, and you actually showered and combed your hair before going out? Just because you live under the same roof doesn't mean you can't make yourself look that good again. Show some respect! Get with it!

- *Dress for success.* If you expect her to wear that black lace teddy you bought for Valentine's Day, the least you can do is wear something that turns her on. Could be a flowered silk shirt, a cashmere sweater, that bikini underwear with a snorting bull embroidered on the front—whatever gets her jazzed.

- *Pop some porn into the VCR.* How many of us grew up without stolen glances at Hef's latest centerfold? These days, pornography of all kinds has moved almost into the mainstream (depending on who you ask—some would argue it's all Hollywood does). What once was mostly close-ups of the old in-out is today a variety of soft to hard porn, some directed by women and aimed at couples. Obviously, this isn't something you push on an unwilling partner, but it might be something to consider.

Enjoy the Sounds of Sex

There's no doubt that sound can be sexy—what else keeps all those 900 numbers in business? These ideas will keep ears ringing and her lust burning:

- *Get rid of distractions.* Again, you want the environment to be conducive to lovemaking. Unplug the phone, turn off your pager, turn down the answering machine. If you're into mood music, keep it soft and choose something you both will enjoy that's not too obtrusive. Stow the Sinatra or Beastie Boys unless you know they're winners.

- *Talk sexy.* There are plenty of ways that talking can enhance foreplay. Simply tell your partner how attracted you are to her, how much you want to make love to her. Chances are this would be welcome—researchers have found that most women want more talk about feelings and affection from their partner during foreplay. Some couples like to taunt and tease each other by talking about the mind-blowing erotic plans they have. Some couples get turned on by "talking dirty," by using slang that expresses desire most directly. Remember, often it's not the words you say, but how you say it, or what your hands are doing at the time.

- *Sound out.* Erotic sounds, whether they're moans of pleasure or murmurs of excitement, can spice up foreplay. When something feels good, don't keep it a secret. And encourage her to do the same.

Touch For Success

What's the body's biggest sex organ? The skin. Our sense of touch is central to being turned on. Here are some ways to make that work for you.

- *Undress for success.* You've already undressed her with your eyes. Now do it with your hands. One study found that 90% of the women surveyed were excited by a man gently and seductively disrobing them. We already know you don't have to be talked into it.

- *Know her zones.* Everybody has their own preferences when it comes to touching. Genitals and breasts are obvious sexual hot spots, but don't neglect eyelids, ears, shoulders, feet, neck, face, palms, inner thighs. Not only are some areas of her body more sensitive than others, the same area might respond differently to a light touch, a gentle stroke or a firm massage. And a touch may elicit one reaction at the beginning of lovemaking and a different one in the throes of passion. Consider it your mission to explore and discover her favorite combinations. It may take several expeditions to map all this out, but you're up to it, right?

- *Spark, then smolder.* Good foreplay, especially touch, starts slowly and builds to a crescendo. And it doesn't move in a straight line from A to B. The best plan of attack involves advancing, retreating, advancing a little farther, retreating again, and so on, until you're both so crazed with desire that the windows are steamed shut.

Pleasures of the G Spot

Maybe you've heard people refer to it but have never used its power to turbocharge foreplay. If so, here's the low down on the G spot so you can add it to your list of favorites for turning her on.

The female G spot is an area located on the forward wall of the vagina, under the urethra, roughly halfway in (its location, and even its existence, is disputed by some). Many women experience deep pleasure from it being touched by fingers or penis (a steady pressure generally seems more stimulating than rubbing). A variation would be to stimulate her G spot with one finger and her clitoris with your thumb.[64]

The prostate gland has been called the male G spot, because of its sensitivity and role in orgasm. It can be stimulated by pressure on your perineum, the area between your testicles and anus.

Not everyone responds to or even acknowledges either the male or female G spot. Why not experiment and decide for yourself?

Taste: How Sweet It Is

Your tongue is good for more than just talking. Again, use your tongue in an advance-and-retreat move, becoming increasingly intimate and arousing as you go. Why not try a dollop of strawberry jam on her breasts, paired, perhaps, with some peanut butter elsewhere? And remember, the last thing she wants to taste when you kiss her is the salami on rye you had for lunch—so keep your breath fresh with strategic brushing, flossing, mouth-wash, breath mints, or whatever it takes. For information on foods that may enhance sexual experiences, see *Aphrodisiacs*.

Many couples enjoy oral stimulation of the clitoris and/or penis. For an extended discussion of these pleasures, see the *Oral Sex* chapter.

Smell: Last But Not Least

Women are generally more sensitive than men to smells, which means she may be able to tell that you haven't bathed since Thursday even though you think you're fresh as a daisy. So hit the showers—cologne won't cover up your stink once you're in a clinch. Everyone has scents they prefer, and those they avoid, but research suggests that some surprising scents may have universal effects. One study reported that lavender and pumpkin best boosted male arousal—as measured by blood flow to the genitals—while women were most aroused by the smell of Good & Plenty candy and cucumbers.[65] Will those smells work the same way on you and your lover? Maybe not, but they may be a good place to start exploring erotic aromas.

FOREPLAY FOR YOU

Contrary to what you might think, women aren't mind readers. She may not always know what turns you on. How do you ask for what you want without coming across like Mr. Selfish?

- *Don't just put up with it.* Not telling your partner that something does-n't feel good is dishonest, and doesn't help anyone. If you don't speak up, she might have no idea that you'd like something done differently.
- *Pick the right time.* Often the best time to talk about sex isn't when you're about to start, in the middle, or just finished. It's too easy for your comments to sound like criticism. Try to hear your comments from her point of view, and find a time for them, when she's most open—certainly not in an argument.

- *Set an example.* Let her know that any time she'd like you to do something differently, she should tell you. If she knows you're open to change, she'll feel less threatened when you make suggestions to her.
- *Talk about yourself.* Not that you should be self-centered. But when you describe what "I'm feeling," or what "I like," you're not focusing attention on what she's doing wrong or not doing right. Talking in the first person will tend to keep things gentler and less accusatory—and better for both of you.
- *Give feedback.* Many women not only want you to tell them what you're feeling during foreplay, they find it arousing. Simple phrases like "that feels good," or "a little harder (or softer)" will help her give you what you want.

OUTERCOURSE: WHEN FOREPLAY REIGNS

Men like foreplay. In fact, most of the men surveyed for the Hite study said that they greatly enjoyed feeling aroused for a long period of time before orgasm. But the same study also found that most men expect foreplay to lead to intercourse. The truth is, sex can be whatever you and your partner define it to be. That might mean spending the evening passionately kissing and touching each other. It might mean giving each other an erotic massage, or giving each other orgasms orally. Outercourse—sex with anything but intercourse—can:

- Allow you to pleasure each other without fear of pregnancy, when contraception is unavailable or inconvenient.
- Reduce tension. Once coitus is off the agenda, there's less pressure to perform. The usual script has been thrown out and suddenly you're both free to improvise.
- Add variety. Finding yourself in a sexual rut? Enjoy the erotic meandering of non-coital sex. Pleasures you may have underestimated can bloom into deeply satisfying moments, drawing you surprisingly close to your partner and producing undreamed of satisfaction for both of you.

Whether outercourse or intercourse is more appropriate is determined by the desire and drives of the moment and the two people involved.

GROOMING

Like it or not, you're a walking advertisement for yourself.

And here's the message your grooming habits convey: "This is who I am...this is my level of self-esteem...this is how much I care about style, cleanliness, and my appearance to others..."

Of course some people read other messages as well, such as "So that's his level of ambition, his savvy and well-being, his class, his..." well, it never ends, and at some point you need to make some basic decisions about your image. For better or worse, who we are and how we look are irrevocably bound. What do you advertise about yourself through grooming?

Some men couldn't care less. A quarter-inch stubble, old tee shirt, and a grubby pair of work boots is their take-it-or-leave-it statement. For others it's an Armani suit and the perfect tie. Hey, different strokes for different blokes. Professions often determine a required level of grooming. So can a concern with how we look to the ladies.

Of course the message we intend to send is not always the message received. And the message she receives is what concerns us here. Bad breath, wire-brush whiskers, or an inflamed blackhead can make a resounding statement before we get a chance to speak.

Grooming is about image, health, and sexual fitness (you may consider yourself fit and all ready for sex; your grooming may be saying something else entirely).

So here's a head-to-toe survey for how to keep your outer self hale and healthy. Use it to get to first base. Then turn on the charm and head for extra bases and sexual glory.

SAVE YOUR SKIN

Fortunately, skin requires remarkably little maintenance given its demanding job of acting as your first line of defense against the outside world. Generally speaking, men are less concerned with the condition of their skin than women. Still, men's toiletries is a multibillion-dollar industry today, and a substantial portion of that goes to skin care.

Are you thick-skinned? The truth is, your skin varies in thickness, ranging from 1.5 millimeters (on hands and feet) to .05 (eyelids).[66] The top layer of your skin, the epidermis, continuously sends new skin cells upward that die and eventually flake off. This produces the beautifully regenerating, mostly non-scarring surface you present to the world. Here's how to keep it in tip-top shape.

Nine Tips for Healthy Skin

1. *Be smart about the sun.* Wrinkles, age spots, sun burn, and skin cancer can all be consequences of sun exposure. No, you don't have to become nocturnal. But you should avoid prolonged sun exposure when possible, especially from 10 to 3. If you can't, use a sunscreen and wear a wide-brimmed hat. You're better off not trying to tan, but if you must, use a sunscreen that offers an SPF of 15 or more (and put it on at least 20 minutes before you head outdoors) and shields against both U-V-A and U-V-B radiation. Reconsider tanning salons. Tune into your local weather forecast—depending on your location, it may give you the new ultraviolet index for the coming day so you can plan your outdoor activities accordingly.

   Remember, some people start to sunburn after only 10 minutes in direct sunlight. If you use Retin-A an anti-aging skin care, be doubly sure you use sunscreen. Like other medications (some antibiotics, anti-histamines, etc.), it can increase your skin's photosensitivity dramatically.

2. *Don't smoke.* Besides the obvious health hazards you've already heard about, smoking is also believed to make your skin thinner.

3. *Drink plenty of water*—anywhere from eight glasses to half your body weight in ounces per day. Your skin needs water and you have to supply it. Drink all through the day—don't wait until you're thirsty. And don't depend on drinks with caffeine for your water needs; they can increase rather than decrease your body's water needs.

4. *Choose a shower over a bath* when possible if you're troubled by dry, itchy skin. Sure, it's nice to lie down and soak in warm water, but you can wash away your skin's protective oils. Dermatologists at the University of Texas Southwestern Medical Center advise a quick shower and warm, rather than hot, water.[67] When you get out, pat yourself dry but leave your skin moist. Since dry skin is a matter of low water content, moisturizers help by locking moisture in—oil on dry skin won't help. Moisturizing lotions, with emulsifiers that keep oil and

water mixed, are the real-world alternative to overly oily, but wonderfully protective, products like petroleum jelly.

5. *Don't overdo the soap.* It too can strip skin's protective oils. Men with oily skin can regulate the level of oils on their skin by using more or less soap.

Getting Hip Safely

Thinking about getting a tattoo or having your tongue pierced? Make sure you see sterilized or disposable (one-use) tools. Otherwise you're putting yourself at risk for pesky infections or serious diseases like Hepatitis B/C or AIDS.

---

6. *Win the battle against dust mites.* A daily morning shower could be just the thing to minimize the effects of the microscopic creatures in your bedding that can cause skin irritations.

7. *Take action on acne.* If you haven't outgrown acne, you're not alone—millions of people have the adult version. The best approach is simple: wash your face gently with a mild soap (washing too often or too vigorously can make it worse). Seek out an over-the-counter medication that's designed for adults, or see a dermatologist if adult acne persists.

8. *Consider cosmetic surgery.* Men are increasingly accepting the high expense of reversing sagging skin and wrinkles (facelifts, dermabrasion, chemical peels), drooping eyelids (blepharoplasty), going for nose jobs (rhinoplasty), and/or fat removal (liposuction). Pros and cons of each are discussed during your initial consultation—find a reputable surgeon through the American Board of Plastic Surgery at (800) 635-0635.

9. *Splash on some cologne.* Some women love it. In fact, some women are turned on by it. A recent study showed that two days after the end of menstruation, women were more sexually aroused in the presence of cologne.[68] But the reverse was true in the middle of their cycle. Timing is everything.

Five Steps to the Perfect Shave

Whose idea was it for men to start their days by sliding an intensely sharp object across their faces? Well, now it's the look, so unless you avoid the ritual with a beard, remember the foundation of a great shave: good prep and good blade.[69]

- *Soak and soften.* For a memorable shave, soften your face and whiskers with a sink of very warm (but not uncomfortably hot) water, soap, and a wash cloth (if you've never actually used a wet towel or washcloth, do yourself a favor and try it). Press the cloth against your face for a minute or two to soften whiskers and melt away any residual stress you still feel from dreams of being chased by your boss. Feels good, yes?

   For a dry shave, the prep is the same, but complete it by drying your face and applying shaving powder.

- *Lather up.* For shaving wet, apply shaving cream, gel, or soap evenly, with circular motions, working all areas of skin to be shaved.

- *Begin shaving* the easiest parts of your beard first (saving the tough parts for later gives the hairs more time to soften). *Always shave in the direction the hair grows*—it's easier on your skin. Discover the grain of your beard by rubbing your fingers across your whiskers. Going with the grain feels smooth; against the grain feels rough. [Note: shave against the grain with an electric razor, using small circles with circular blades.]

- *Shave* with short, easy strokes and rinse your razor every few passes. Carefully lift the blade off your face after each stroke to minimize nicks.

- *Rinse well* when you're done, using the washcloth, unless you prefer invigorating splashes. Pat, don't wipe—your skin's taken enough of a beating already. Use a moisturizer to soothe and keep your skin supple. If over-dryness is a problem, avoid alcohol-based aftershaves. Go natural with aloe vera gel, nature's burn-relief aftershave.

CARE FOR HAIR

Once upon a time, men's grooming consisted of a shave and haircut. Now more and more men are going for color, curls, transplants, and other embellishments. Again, it may be vanity or it may be a necessary tool for your job. Here are some hair-care options.

- *Treat it gently when wet.* Wet hair is more easily damaged, so don't brush or rub it roughly when it's wet. If it's hard to manage, use a conditioner after shampooing.

- *Read directions for shampoos and conditioners.* More is not necessarily better. Using a hair care product improperly can turn your mane brittle. Ditto for coloring, bleaches, etc. Shampooing every day is okay unless your hair is extra dry.

- *Don't over-brush.* Brushing or combing too much can be damaging, so don't work it more than you need to. Avoid sharp-tipped brushes and fine-toothed combs.

- *Differentiate hair loss from balding.* Losing up to 100 hairs a day is normal, but if you think your hair loss is excessive, see a dermatologist.[70] Receding hair is common—over 60% of men develop some sort of balding as they age. Hereditary baldness can come from either the mother's or father's side of the family. There is no cure for balding, but some forms of hair loss can be treated by hair transplantation or prescription medication.

- *Treat dandruff.* Dead hair flaking off your scalp is normal. But when dandruff becomes an evident problem, take action. First, simply try daily shampooing. If that isn't enough, move up to shampoos with zinc pyrithionate. Allow 3-4 weeks and if you don't notice improvement, try a shampoo containing selenium sulfide or salicylic acid. Then it's on to products with tar. Beyond that it's cortisone-containing lotions or creams, which can cause side effects, and so should be used with care. Talk to your doctor if none of the above solutions work.

DON'T FORGET YOUR NAILS

Made mostly of the protein keratin, nails are more than just what you think of as a toenail or fingernail—they're a system of parts working together. The plate is the most obvious; under it is the nail bed. The matrix, under the cuticle, is where the nail grows from. Together, these parts can tell a doctor a lot about the health of your heart, liver, lungs, etc.

Keeping your nails clean not only looks good, it prevents bacteria and other nasty stuff from setting up shop and causing more serious, painful, or ugly problems. Once again, beauty is in the eye of the beholder, so just because you don't care about your nails, don't think she won't.

- *Avoid ingrown nails.* When one corner of a nail grows down and into your skin, you may need medical help to avoid infection. Avoid that problem to begin with by proper nail trimming and shoes that fit properly.

- *Trim your nails*   straight across the fingertip and round the edges slightly to keep them strong and from growing into your skin.

- *Soak your toenails*   in warm salt water for five to ten minutes if they're too thick to clip. You can also use commercially-available urea cream to help soften them for trimming.

CARE FOR YOUR TEETH AND SMILE

False teeth may have been fine for George Washington, but you're better off keeping your choppers in good working order. Regular dental care keeps bacteria called plaque from roosting in your mouth, attacking tooth enamel, and sending you to the dentist's chair to endure one of life's truly awful experiences: cavity drilling. Act now to avoid it!

- *Brush twice a day.*   Hold your toothbrush at a 45-degree angle and move it gently back and forth or in small circles ending with a gentle stroke down. Remember to cover the outer tooth surfaces, the inner tooth surfaces, and the chewing surfaces of the teeth. Use fluoride toothpaste.

- *Floss or use other between-the-teeth cleaners.*   Ask your dentist about the right technique for you.

- *Change your toothbrush every three months.*   You don't want to know about the bacteria that's taken up residence on that toothbrush. Also worn bristles don't clean as efficiently and can hurt your gums.

FRESHEN YOUR BREATH

You lean in to kiss her. She pulls a gas mask out of her purse. You've got halitosis—or, as it's more commonly known, dog breath. Don't worry, a few simple precautions can usually tame it.

- *Brush and floss regularly.*   If the the prospect of eating all your meals with a straw isn't enough to get you to appreciate good dental hygiene, maybe the fact that your breath smells like rotting food should do it.

- *Brush your tongue*   when you finish brushing your teeth. Food particles that get stuck there are magnets for odor-causing bacteria.

- *Avoid tobacco* like the poison it is. Consider the consequences of moving in for your first kiss smelling like an ashtray.

- *Use mouthwashes and breath fresheners in a pinch,* but don't depend on them. They may mask the odor but they don't treat the cause. And if certain foods like garlic are the cause, the odor is coming from your lungs so brushing alone won't help.

- *Treat dry mouth and sinus problems.* Both can contribute to halitosis. Ask your doctor what will work for you.

BODY ODOR

Everybody has BO thanks to bacteria that live on your body and like warm, moist places like your armpits. The more you sweat, the happier, and smellier, they become. Before your aroma gets out of hand:

- *Bathe regularly.* Duh, right? But hey, if you're so smart, how come you stink? Regular baths or showers get rid of both sweat and bacteria.

- *Use antibacterial soap.* It's like a smart bomb that wipes out those stinky germs.

- *Try every option.* Some underarm products are deodorants—they kill bacteria and mask odors. Others are antiperspirant—they stop up sweat glands. Some products do both. Choose a product with the scent, or lack thereof, that most appeals to you.

- *Talk to your doctor.* There are prescription products that can help severe cases.

HORMONES

Ask a man what hormones do. He'll probably tell you they drive him nuts once a month. What he means, of course, is that he's affected by the mood swings his wife or girlfriend experiences in her menstrual cycle, which is driven in part by hormonal activity.

He may also mention the much-debated estrogen replacement therapy many women now use to offset the reduction of that primarily female hormone during and after menopause.

But what he's less likely to mention, because it's a relatively new topic, or because he prefers not to consider it, is how *his own* hormones affect *him*. The topic of men and hormones has expanded beyond those men who take steroids to enhance their athletic performance. Nowadays there's much discussion about how hormones affect a man's day-to-day moods, his performance at work and in family life, his health and fitness, how he ages and whether he can slow that process considerably with hormone replacement therapy of his own.

And one other related subject that might interest him—and you—is the dramatic influence hormones have on male sexual potency, desire and performance.

HORMONES AND YOU

Hormones are swift chemical messengers that control how you react to minute-to-minute living. They're part of your endocrine system, a network of glands that produce hormones and other biochemicals.

Those endocrine glands—your own pharmaceutical factories—create hormones and send them into your bloodstream, where they circulate to whatever part of your body needs to respond to stimulation. For example, when you eat, insulin (a hormone) is released to help convert food to the fuel your muscles need to work. Or when a guy wanders into a topless bar, the gyrating visual stimulation he gets can produce a surge of the male sex hormone testosterone,[71] about which we'll have more to say shortly.

Your body produces and uses many hormones on a daily basis. They function as emergency high-priority messengers, painkillers, and tranquilizers, among other functions. Let's take a quick overview of those, and then plunge into sex hormones.

Probably the most dramatic human physiological reaction is the flight-or-fight response. You'll find more about it in the *Stress* chapter, but since it's a hormonal response, we'll briefly describe it here. In short, all systems are put on high alert to deal with a perceived threat. The hormone adrenaline is pumped into the bloodstream to prepare the heart, respiratory system, and muscles for extreme action, either to fight for food or defense, or to flee danger. Wonderful when a wild animal ambushes you in a gully. But modern threats like office politics or financial worries provoke the same response. In time, the cardiovascular system becomes stressed and can be damaged without appropriate exercise or other de-stressing solutions. Chronic anxiety, about sex or otherwise, can therefore take a serious toll on health.

Biochemical painkillers called endorphins produce the famous runner's high. And biotranquilizers like melotonin and serotonin calm and equalize. Then there's the sex hormones.

MAKE WAY FOR TESTOSTERONE

Although it plays a role in metabolism, strength, growth, bone density and more, testosterone is best known as the primary male sex hormone. Produced in the gonads and the adrenal gland, its influence first occurs in the womb, where at the proper time it produces male characteristics, such as a penis. Its next big impact is in adolescence, when it initiates puberty. A deficiency of testosterone production in the testes, called hypogonadism, can delay puberty and cause other developmental problems. Doctors intervene with testosterone replacement, a therapy not without risk because of possible adverse reactions if too much of the hormone is administered. Hypogonadism is not restricted to boys, for whom genetics may be the cause. Men can also suffer from it by disease or injury. Symptoms can include decreased sex drive and sperm count[72] or impotence.[73] When a blood test reveals low testosterone, one answer is simply to add more.

Testosterone can be replaced in three basic ways: pills, patches, or injections.[74] Since the hormone's natural production and transmission occur in cycles throughout the day, the aim of testosterone replacement therapy is to mimic that delivery as closely as possible. Pills and injections don't do that as well as dermal patches, which were once worn only on the scrotum, but newer versions offer more comfort and convenience. When used properly the therapy restores normal sexual functioning.

But there are dangers. If too much testosterone is introduced, the risk of prostate enlargement or cancer increases. Caution is advised, especially

**Symptoms Of Low
Testosterone:**[76]

- less energy, strength, or muscle tone
- erection problems
- decreased sexual desire
- increased irritability
- slower facial hair growth
- breast enlargement
- scrotum shrinkage
- profuse sweating

for any man with cancer. Also, research has shown that prostate tests can fail to show early cancer in men with low testosterone levels.[75] If you're considering testosterone replacement, ask your doctor about having a biopsy done first to be extra safe.

In case you're wondering, testosterone replacement therapy is not a miracle sex booster for normal men and may only create the risks described above.

Low testosterone levels can be measured by a simple blood test. See your doctor for details.

THE AGE OF ANTI-AGING

Testosterone is also being used to reverse one of the basic conditions known to mankind—aging. The basis of this practice proceeds from the fact that certain hormones usually tend to decrease in men when they are in their 40's. Not as dramatically as in women in menopause, but dramatically enough for some to be talking about male menopause. In fact, women's hormone replacement therapy (HRT) together with new male HRT has produced one of the newest areas of medical practice: anti-aging.

DHEA

Another hormone that boosts sex drive is dehydroepiandrosterone, or DHEA. Although known since the 30's, this hormone has received much attention in this decade because of research demonstrating its capacity to boost energy, promote sleep, and help relax and neutralize stress.[77] Some researchers cite the decrease of DHEA in a man's thirties as part of male menopause, and accept its role as a sex drive stimulator.[78]

Naturally produced in the adrenal gland, it is currently available without a prescription in pills synthesized from Mexican wild yams. Typical studies suggest that those with low levels of DHEA benefit from its replacement, while those with normal levels do not. Like testosterone, long-term HRT studies with DHEA are only getting started now, so long-term safety is not confirmed. The best person to ask about using it would be your doctor.

Anti-Aging Comes of Age

As the Baby Boom generation advances into middle age, more Americans than ever before will be looking, like Ponce de León in the Florida wilderness, for a fountain of youth. And they'll find an unprecedented variety of solutions—clinics, books, newsletters, products, physicians, therapies, and more. Here are a few resources for the latest news:

- National Association for Human Development: (202) 328-2192
- National Council on the Aging: (202) 479-1200
- The Rejuvenation and Longevity Foundation: www.anti-aging.org
- Aging Research Center: www.arclab.org
- American Academy of Anti-Aging: www.worldhealth.net

Hormone replacement is one anti-aging option among others. As we've seen there are risks, but doctors who advocate the practice say their goal is only to return hormone levels to where they once were, and not more. Dr. Randall Urban, a Texas endocrinologist, found in a small study that while testosterone replacement did increase strength and sex drive in some, he still thinks exercise (specifically strength-training) is a better alternative until more tests are done.[79] He currently regards anti-aging testosterone replacement therapy as best for men in their 80's.

IMPOTENCE
(ERECTILE DYSFUNCTION)

Impotence. Not many words strike such fear into the hearts of men. No wonder a new term—erectile dysfunction, or ED—is replacing it. The newer version has a more abstract and, well, softer sound, with less history stacked on its shoulders. It makes the problem sound less like a stigma than a treatable condition, which it is.

That's great news for the men who suffer in its shadow. Dr. Ken Goldberg, author of *How Men Can Live As Long As Women*, estimates that 30 million American men are impotent[80]. One in four! That's a whole lot of anguish. The good news today is that no man should resign himself to sitting on the sidelines of the sensual pleasures of sex. All should—and can— enjoy the thrill and deep satisfaction it brings. In fact, no man should shrink from what ED ultimately is—a challenge, like any other. If this is a problem for you, explore it wholeheartedly as with any other problem in your life, and have faith that you will emerge into the warm light of a satisfying sex life again.

Whether you call it impotence or ED, the definition is the same: consistently unable to achieve or maintain an erection for satisfying intercourse. Most men experience it at some point in their lives. There are many different causes and many different treatments and we'll examine them all—yes, including the mighty Viagra. Our first step is to revisit what makes an erection happen, and not happen, and then we'll get to what makes it happily happen again.

A QUICK LOOK INSIDE

Romance aside, an erection is about blood, nerves, and smooth muscle tissue. We'll summarize the process here, which is covered in more detail in the *Penis* chapter.

An erection usually begins in the brain, which sends nerve signals to the penis, setting off several physiological events which produce the desired stiffness. The interior of the penis consists largely of spongy tissue. The nerve signals make that tissue relax, which allows penile arteries to expand with blood. As they expand they constrict veins which temporarily cut off the outflow of blood from the penis. Through hydraulic action, the penis rises, gets hard, and stands ready for glorious action.

There are emotional as well as physical reasons for ED. Though that sounds neat and tidy, the fact is that the two can overlap. For example, if a man suffers ED due to a medication he takes, he can feel anxious about trying to make love. That anxiety produces physical reactions of its own, which con-

> **The Essence of an Erection**
>
> When blood flows freely in and out of a penis, it stays soft.
>
> When blood flows in but is blocked from flowing out—bango!—stiff penis.

tribute to his faltering confidence. Correcting his medication can be a simple solution, as long as his anxiety doesn't stand in his way, in which case that needs to be addressed. Sounds complicated, but it doesn't have to be. Now let's take a more detailed look at the reasons and then get to the solutions.

EIGHT COMMON CAUSES OF ERECTION PROBLEMS

Fatigue

Many men today feel they must be able to make love at all times in all places. Hey, maybe a reluctant penis is telling you something! If you're too tired for sex, why not accept that? There's no need to question your manhood. ED is a tough way to learn that lesson, but it is a clear one.

Stress

When survival was at stake historically, either in the moment, as with a sudden intruder, or in troubled times of drought or famine, sex and procreation moved off center stage. Adrenaline, the hormone that initiates emergency bodily changes, works against the normal mechanics of an erection. So do the effects of longer term stress: headaches, depression, high blood pressure, asthma, arthritis, stomach pain, digestive disorders, diarrhea, frequent colds, and much more. Healthy sex is an expression of love and intimacy, but its foundation is a fit body and mind. Long-term stress undermines both, and should be neutralized ASAP with appropriate lifestyle changes.

Ailments and Conditions

Cardiovascular disease and diabetes are leading causes of ED. Anything that restricts the flow of blood to or in the penis, such as high blood pressure, high cholesterol, and clogging of the arteries, works against an erection. A cholesterol test can help determine if those are a factor in impotence. If so, several natural remedies are available to help, exercise being at the top of the list. As a remedy of last resort, penile bypass surgery is available for correcting serious artery blockages. Diabetes can be a factor too, affecting both blood flow and nerves. Your doctor can tell you about other conditions that might be of relevance to you.

Medications

The publicity about deaths from Viagra has put a new spotlight on the dangers of medical drugs. But adverse reactions to medications aren't new—ED is a side effect of many drugs used either in combination or alone. For instance, heart disease medication can make a man twice as likely to suffer from ED.[81] And complicating the picture even more is the fact that one medication can be a problem for one man and not for another. Common sense and observation, plus input from your doctor, is the answer. Besides switching medications, you can also ask your doctor about the implications of reducing your dosage. A list of specific drugs—antihypertensives, antidepressants, and more—can be found in *Medications*.

Hormones

A man may have read an ad about testosterone replacement therapy and be convinced he needs it. And he might. But it's not nearly as common a cause of ED as others listed here. A simple test can answer the question. Besides aging, high on the list of probable hormone-related erectile difficulties are testicular disease and alcoholism.

Alcohol

Research has confirmed that moderate drinking is good for your health, right? Well, yes, some studies have shown that up to two drinks a day (one for women) can be good for your arteries. And as we've seen, what's good for your arteries is good for your sex life. The picture is not totally rosy, however; moderate alcohol consumption has also been associated with raised blood pressure.[82] The benefits disappear with heavy drinking. And while age is the number one contributing factor for high blood pressure, a recent study shows that when young, healthy men were "exposed acutely" to alcohol, their bloodstream testosterone levels dropped consistently.[83]

Tobacco

The chemistry of tobacco smoke meeting cholesterol is bad news for blood vessels. Once healthy arteries become in time constricted and inelastic, clogged with plaque, and restricting the health-promoting flow of blood, including vessels in the penis. Cigarettes also cause something called vaso-constriction, which amounts to the same thing: narrowed arteries, which in the penis can be caused by just two cigarettes.[84]

Negative Emotions

ED is never a laughing matter, but it hits especially hard for someone who is already depressed, or filled with anxiety about his ability to "perform." Plus, those emotions, along with frustration and anger, can all too easily follow problems with physical causes, and remain after the physical problems have been successfully treated. If the emotions persist, and talking with your partner or doctor doesn't help, seeing a sex therapist can often provide a breakthrough. More on that below.

> **ED Emotional First-aid**
> Don't panic. Acknowledge what happened; don't deny it. Seek answers and support. Change attitudes if necessary (you as sex machine may have to change to human being). Relax. Have faith in yourself.

GOOD NEWS: SIX TREATMENTS THAT WORK

Until recently, treatment for ED consisted mostly of counselling, chemical injections, hormone therapy, implants, or surgery. Then came Viagra! The other treatments still have their place, and we'll look at them, but we'll start by looking at the "wonder pill."

Viagra

Spring, 1998: Doctors use rubber stamped prescriptions to keep up with demand...men scurry over the border to obtain pills not approved in Canada...blanket media coverage...VIP's admitting their delight...what a buzz!

As the dust settles, research will reveal the verdict on the Viagra phenomenon. On one side are millions of men with new ability and enthusiasm for sex. On the other side are doctors and regulatory agencies nervously reading reports of deaths associated with its use.

In fact, at about the 6 million prescription mark, the FDA revised its labelling requirement with new safety warnings. But that didn't substantially diminish the interest in sildenafil, the active ingredient causing the stir. Clearly, many men like having a cure for ED as close as their local drug store.

Viagra produces an erection by prolonging the effects of a chemical called cyclic GMP, which allows the penis to fill with blood and stay filled long enough for satisfying intercourse. The pill is prescribed for once a day, from 30 minutes to 4 hours before intercourse. Side effects are relatively mild: headaches, flushing, upset stomach, stuffy nose, urinary tract infection, blue-tinged vision, and diarrhea.

But those are not the side effects that most concerned the FDA. It was the 130 fatal heart attacks suffered while using Viagra (in America). While not affirming that the new medication was the cause of those deaths, the FDA and Pfizer, the drug's manufacturer, changed the warning label to include:[85]

- Reports of heart attacks, sudden cardiac deaths, and high blood pressure.
- Advising men with preexisting cardiovascular conditions that use of Viagra carries enhanced risk.
- Warnings regarding the risk of lowered blood pressure while using the drug.
- Noting that the clinical trials of Viagra did not include patients with cardiovascular problems.
- Advising patients with prolonged erections (longer than 4 hours) to seek immediate medical attention.

There's an important message there that definitely applies to Viagra, but goes beyond it too—namely, that ED is often a signal of cardiovascular conditions that demand attention. Therefore before taking Viagra, you should undergo a thorough medical exam. Because ED could be a warning signal of other physical problems, it should not be ignored. Lastly, with Viagra there is a danger in ignoring an emotional aspect of ED and in not exploring the depths of intimacy which might itself bring drug-free relief and new satisfaction.

That said, one certainly has to cheer for all the men who have experienced renewed pleasure from sex. As to the possible side effects, time will have to tell.

Suddenly many older ED treatments look a lot less attractive. But not to men who would rather not take the small statistical risk of new impotence pills, or to those for whom they don't work. Alternatives follow.

Injections

Some drugs create an erection independent of arousal, which is different from sildenafil (Viagra), which like a natural erection requires the release of nitric oxide via the central nervous system. The traditional drawback was that they require an injection from a small needle into the base of the penis. Side effects include an erection lasting more than 4 hours—which is dangerous—dizziness, and possible liver damage. Self-injections are also relatively expensive.

Implants

This is a surgical option which places a semirigid or inflatable prosthesis inside the penis, creating an erection independent of blood flow. Semirigid implants are rods which are simply bent straight for an erection, and then back into a curve for a "flaccid" state. In actuality, the penis is always semi-erect. But the device is simpler in practice than injections. Inflatable implants are more complicated, with more chance of necessary repair, but are more natural when soft than the semirigid type. Both replace natural tissue without which a natural erection is not possible.

Vacuum Devices

Vacuum devices produce an erection by bringing blood into the penis and trapping it there. A plastic tube is placed over the penis and a vacuum created by a small hand pump draws blood into the penis. Then a soft ring is placed around the base of the penis to keep the blood from draining back into the body. This method doesn't have the disadvantages or side effects of implants and injections, but disrupts the flow of sex. The penis ring must be removed within 30 minutes to avoid damaging tissue by restrained blood flow.

Yohimbine

Derived from an African tree bark, yohimbine is the standardized, prescription form of the herb yohimbe. It works by stimulating the nervous system. Because it also reputably stimulates sexual desire, it bridges the gap between the medical treatments previously discussed and the scientifically-unvalidated area of aphrodisiacs. But that doesn't invalidate the enthusiasm reported by satisfied users. Mild side effects like dizziness, irritability and nausea have been reported.

Sex Therapy

Don't think of it as endlessly rehashing your childhood. A sex therapist will work with specific problems toward specific goals. Starting the process—getting over the hurdle of not being able to talk about ED—is a major step forward. The course of treatment usually includes exercises done at home, and progress can build after only a few sessions. A sex therapist is also trained to know when to work with a doctor when medications or mechanical devices might prove temporarily useful. To some it might sound trite, but certainly not to those who have experienced it: sex therapy can open doors to territory men didn't even know existed. More than just dealing with problems, sex therapy can expand a man's sex life to a sense of fulfillment and happiness never before imagined.

IMPOTENCE IN THE WORLD

After seven years of marriage and a divorce, Bill found a new job in a new city. Then he met Tina at work. They had been dating for a month when one Friday night, after a movie, she invited him for a nightcap in her apartment. He had begun to wonder if they were right for each other, but when she suggested getting in bed he thought why not, maybe this will shed some light on the situation. It did. He was between Tina's legs, ready to enter her, when his erection disappeared. She turned her face away. Bill didn't know what to say so he said nothing. He had never experienced this before. Tina asked him to try again, but he couldn't keep an erection long enough to get inside her. She said maybe it was time for this fiasco of an evening to end. He dressed and left feeling like half a man and a total failure. They had a quick conversation the next day in which Tina suggested they not see each other any more.

Bill didn't date for a year. He felt slightly reassured that he could still masturbate, but didn't even feel comfortable enough bringing up his problem with his brothers. Then he was introduced to Jill. They met for coffee a few times, and then started dating. Needless to say, he was nervous about sex. She sensed it and made him feel comfortable, kissing and touching him. When they finally went to bed together it happened again. This time *he* turned away, his mind reeling with despair. But she told him not to worry, and held him tight until he turned back. They talked for awhile and then she held his penis until it stiffened and then guided it inside her. Bill felt like he was in heaven. Over the next few weeks he realized that he hadn't really been attracted in any deep way to Tina. With Jill he felt a connection stronger than his anxiety about performing. But even with Jill he would occasionally try to make love when he wasn't really into it, and would fail. He was learning that trying to make love when he wasn't feeling the desire was a mistake, and he gradually felt strong enough to say so. Which wasn't necessary as they made love on a deserted Caribbean beach six months later on the first night of their honeymoon.

INTERCOURSE

It's the ultimate intimacy. A holy consummation. A shock of electric ecstasy. Or a quickie in the powder room.

The grand act of intercourse leads in many directions. It creates profound connection and new life. But for those who ignore safe guidelines, it can lead to death. It can define the state of your body, your head, and your heart, reveal where you've been, and beckon with pleasures beyond imagining.

For women, the act is no less complex. Some hate its patriarchal undertones; others love a tension-relieving ride. Some crave the delivery of semen, while others prefer a vibrator. It can be her ultimate fantasy or ultimate sexual abuse.

From desire to orgasm, hormones to tantra, all the chapters of this book relate to intercourse in one way or another. Peak sexual fitness demands being comfortable with intercourse, and at times, being comfortable without it. To fully taste its power and pleasures, it helps to understand its many faces. We'll go beyond the black and white of it, the should's and had better not's. The assumption here is that you're a mature, responsible adult, interested in what you can do with intercourse—and what intercourse can do for you.

We can see in our own past that intercourse is the best of times and the worst of times, and a whole lot of hubbub in between. Let's open our minds and hearts and spirits and take a plunge into this splendid sexual treasure.

IN AND FEELING GOOD

Intercourse starts, in this book's heterosexual focus, with your penis in her vagina, the union called coitus. From there it can get complicated—but not necessarily. At best, sex is an easy, gratifying flow from desire to arousal to intercourse to afterglow. And at worst, two self-centered people grab for maximum pleasure and minimum involvement. Most of us have known both.

You have to admire the physiology of it—penis and vagina perfect partners in the reproductive drama, both well endowed with nerves connected to pleasure centers in the mind. But how does the clitoris fit in the picture? For many women, it generates the most sensory pleasure, and its stimulation becomes central to orgasm. We'll see how that figures into satisfying intercourse. For that, we'll need specifics.

POSITION YOURSELF FOR PLEASURE

Customized coitus! That's what the various positions of intercourse create—different contact of penis and vagina (with differing sensations for different sizes and shapes); different control for each partner; different use of hands and lips; and differing views of each others' eyes and bodies. The many position options are derived from only three basics: man-on-top, woman-on-top, and side-by-side. An alternative, less gender-based categorization would be standing, sitting, kneeling, and lying, with variations for each. That defusing twist of thought may or may not matter to you, but could be meaningful to her.

Man-on-Top

You're lying above her, between her spread legs. The missionary position delivers big pleasures but has some drawbacks too, as do the others.

On the plus side, there's plenty of skin-to-skin contact. Obviously, you're more in control of your movement and hers in this position. If you like chest to chest contact, you're in the right place. Her face is naturally accessible, so lips and tongues can meet easily. Her arms are free to touch your back, buttocks, and testicles, or wherever your preferences lie. If pregnancy is your goal, this is a blue ribbon position (made even better by raising her hips with a pillow).

The downside of this classic is that it's not the easiest for clitoral stimulation. And sure, you can caress her, but in a limited way since you're supporting your weight with your arms. Men with a tendency toward rapid ejaculation might find more control in positions where less muscular tension is necessary for support. And some women prefer the freedom of movement and control of other positions.

Variations: The angle of her knees significantly changes the relationship of penis and vagina. When her knees are straight, and legs down, her clitoris gets the most stimulation. If she bends her knees, you go deeper, and deeper yet with her legs over your shoulders. Men with shorter penises enjoy that penetration. But remember the advantages of varying the depth of your penetration, and the sensitivity of the outer two inches of her vagina. So tantalize her, and yourself, by alternating between barely in, going deep, and going deepest.

You can also be on top but with her legs together, a position that enhances the stimulation of penis and clitoris.

Woman-On-Top

You're lying on your back and she's sitting or kneeling while straddling your hips, facing you. Your legs can be flat or raised by bent knees. It's a good position for women who want more control over the angle of penile penetration, movement, and/or the general pace of lovemaking, and the best position for men who want more ejaculatory control. She can lean forward to bring her breasts closer to your mouth, or back against your raised thighs, or all the way back between your legs to lean on her hands. When she's on top, it's easy for you, or her, to stimulate her clitoris. The position can reverse the feeling and reality of who's being done. If she's pregnant, she will like having her belly free. And if you're overweight, when you're on the bottom a load will have been lifted from her.

Variations: She moves her legs forward to vary stimulation for both of you. Also, she turns around and faces your legs, which makes it easy for you to stimulate her rear, and for her to stimulate your testicles, perineum, or to grasp the base of your penis to combine masturbation with intercourse.

She can also lie on top, either with her or your legs spread.

Side-By-Side

The most mellow positions for intercourse are when you're both lying on your sides. They are good for intimate, low-key sex, or resting between more vigorous positions, or as the final act in a long night of varied lovemaking. Since neither partner is under the other's weight, this is a good position for prolonged sex. There's high-quality, full-body contact, and you face each other, enabling relaxed gazing into each other's eyes. Genital stimulation is light to moderate for both. Either you or she can raise legs for deeper penetration, but then someone will have limbs under weight so you'll have to keep moving.

Face each other or lie front-to-back in the spoon position. When she's very pregnant she'll appreciate having her belly relaxed and free. When you lie behind her, you can easily caress her belly and all her front erogenous zones—this is a primo position for jolly pregnant sex.

Rear Entry

You're both on your knees and you enter her from behind. Some call it doggy style, and some find it degrading. But there are good reasons to feel otherwise. You can reach around to hold her breasts and give her clitoral stimulation with your fingers. Because you're against her legs, buttocks, and possibly her back, feeling tremendous delight from all that skin contact, enjoying the deep penetration, the stimulation is intense.

While some women don't like the position's animal associations, others are positively turned on by same. As usual, it's strictly a personal call, and one to respect.

Sitting and Standing

She sits on your lap, typically on a bed or chair. The position is long on relaxation and intimacy, but short on stimulation of penis, vagina, and clitoris. Yet as a variation among other positions, especially more energetic ones, sitting intercourse allows for great hugging and kissing, and is good for meditative sex.

Standing intercourse requires strength and stamina, especially when you're the only one standing. If you're strong enough, lift her and support her thighs or buttocks with your hands. Her hands are free to roam, even if yours aren't. This position lends itself to passionate, and/or quick sex. Less demanding are the variations with her standing on one leg (on a support if necessary), with the other still raised, or both of you standing.

All these intercourse positions are only the beginning. The *Kama Sutra*, the Indian book of sex and love, lists literally hundreds. When you and your lover experiment, freely communicating and touching and laughing, then you're no longer trying to improve sex, but merely varying it and finding new ways to nourish an already vibrant sexual relationship.

INTERCOURSE IN CONTEXT

Picturing sexual positions is one thing, but real sex is something else. Most men have vast collections of pornographic images stored in their cranial film vaults. It's always a good idea to make sure they don't interfere with the reality of the present, which is where great intercourse happens.

Passionate sex is different than anxious sex, which is different than bored sex, dutiful sex, and so on. Intercourse will differ accordingly. Also, does a long, interrupted evening lay before you? Or is it morning and almost time to get up when inspiration suddenly rises? Again, if your expectations aren't in sync with hers, intercourse will suffer, if it happens at all.

And don't forget your feelings—or to act on them when appropriate. One study showed approximately 30% of men engage in intercourse not because they want to but because it's expected.[86] It's not unusual for men to have erectile problems when they're not truly interested in intercourse and are just going through the motions. So first make sure you're involved and not doing it for someone else's benefit. If you're clear about that and want to anyway, and it works for both of you, fine. But intercourse should be a unifying, not dividing, experience, with her and within yourself.

Also, ask yourself whether intercourse is appropriate at all. Maybe she's menstruating, or worried about pregnancy, or is too tired. Hey, opportunity knocks! Forget intercourse. Rename foreplay loveplay. Savor kissing and touching as ends in themselves. Enjoy oral sex or mutual masturbation. Have some fun instead of the empty experience that never should have been.

David Schnarch, author of *Passionate Couples*, focuses on developing a mature sexual relationship between two committed, emotionally strong lovers. He advocates a deep intimate connection, and suggests ways to foster it, for example by keeping eyes open during kissing, intercourse, and orgasm. It's first a bit of a shock, then, to come upon his thoughts on how to enjoy f---ing.[87]

Again, it's a matter of context. Sex is dirty and painful when done without regard to your partner's values or wishes. But aggressiveness doesn't have to be inconsiderate. F---ing, as Schnarch describes it, can be tremendously liberating, even elevating. When done within a reciprocal caring relationship, it can transport both partners to the transcendent wilds of sex, where the earth shakes and time stands still. From there you don't return in shame, but rather thankful, impressed, and nourished.

HOW 'BOUT A QUICKIE?

Isn't the very suggestion strictly for the sexual stone age—at least forty or fifty years ago? What about everything men have learned about sensitivity and satisfying their partners? Aren't quickies from a time before men cared, or even knew, about a clitoris? What about everything men have learned about satisfying their partners? What about the guilt?

Whoa, let's slow down a minute. As every man knows, a time comes when he just plain wants in, without the preliminaries. If we can get off our high horse for a moment and think of ourselves as animals—smart and moral ones but animals nonetheless—the urge makes sense. Hey, our "relatives," in the animal kingdom do it fast and easy.

As John Gray points out in *Mars and Venus in the Bedroom*, quickies can be part of a couple's integrating their different natures.[88] Just as men have learned to appreciate the longer and more complex arousal needs of a woman, it's fair that she consider his occasional desire for speed, or those times when desires are mismatched. As long as she's comfortable emotionally and physically accommodating him (certainly a lubricant should be used if needed) the occasional quickie can strengthen, not weaken, their relationship.

PAINFUL INTERCOURSE

Intercourse should bring pleasure, and usually does, but for a woman it can be physically painful, and a concerned man will wonder why. One study found that 40% of women surveyed by a gynecologist experienced at least some pain during sex.[89] Don't be dismissive if your lover mentions it. The majority of complaints are physically-based and treatable. A small percentage of women, however, experience cramped vaginal muscles and benefit from relaxation techniques learned in counseling.

Here are some common complaints that can and should be corrected:[90]

- Infections: Yeast infections and herpes sores can cause stinging and itching in the vagina, and make friction uncomfortable. Medications are available.
- Adverse reactions to contraceptive chemicals or feminine deodorant sprays. Try alternatives.
- Dryness in the vagina due to insufficient excitation or aging. Extend foreplay; lubricate with water-based products or saliva.
- Pelvic pain: felt in deep penetration, may signal serious conditions such as an STD or cyst. Suggest a gynecological exam.

These complaints may not be sexy, but not treating them can lead to more serious conditions with much worse consequences. Show you care. Be involved.

SIX TIPS FOR SUPERCHARGING INTERCOURSE

Vary Positions

Sounds like a no-brainer, but so is falling into a rut of the familiar. Varying positions can be an easy way to enliven sex. But be advised: moving beyond sexual habits can bring up hidden anxieties or conflicts, which successful sexual patterns conveniently cover. Move onward. Be open to the feelings that surface. Chances are they'll surface eventually, perhaps in less manageable ways. And while you're at it, thrill to the added sensations and intimacy that alternative positions can bring. Also vary thrusts, penetration, pressure, duration, and other boredom-busting vehicles of pleasure.

Ask and Listen

Okay, you've heard it before. Communication as a must for sexual fitness is a major theme of this book. Don't fall for the popular myth that passionate intercourse should be wordless. Instead, discover the passion that's fed by requests and fantasies and moans and groans. Sexual communication is unique. Enjoy it!

Go for Seamless Sex

Sure, intercourse can be the throbbing main event. But even so, don't cast the rest of sex in merely supporting roles. Don't make a habit of rushing toward a goal. Enjoy the journey. Just because you're in doesn't mean you can't come out, or get soft and get hard again. Valuing arousal and making sure she's super excited before and during intercourse can lead to super orgasms. Of course, one way to insure that arousal and intercourse are seamless is to make sure she's wet and ready for your penis, so you slip in almost without effort.

Try Tenderness

Everyone has a tender side (although with some it's extremely well hidden). When you show your tender side, in words and touch, her tender side responds, and you can connect in powerful ways. Of course life only in the tender zone lacks spark and sweat and sizzle, which have their own advantages. Revel in it all, and don't get lost in the dopey notion that a man needs to be exclusively rough and tough.

Slip and Slide

A little oil goes a long way in boosting intercourse up the pleasure scale. Try it, or a powder like corn starch, to reduce friction on the skin. Any body-worker knows the necessity of oil for a massage. It allows an entirely different way to interact with skin and muscles. The same applies to intercourse. Lubricants produce a sensuality that makes for a super change of pace. Internally, a lubricant can help low vaginal moisture (water-based products or saliva are recommended when using a condom because oil can cause it to rip or otherwise lose its effectiveness as a sperm barrier).

Do It in the Sand

Or on the balcony. Or in the shower. New locations add spice and an exciting charge to intercourse. Let the sun play upon breasts and balls. Obviously, be discreet. Don't go overboard, just enjoy the occasional change of scenery. Feel the freedom! Feed the passion!

INTIMACY

This chapter examines the greatest sex enhancer of all time: intimacy. Without it, in the long run even the most well-conditioned partners wrestle toward frustration, and technique-centered lovers grope in discontent. Intimacy is the gateway to ultimate sexual satisfaction. And now it's even been linked to increased longevity. Dean Ornish, the maverick doctor who revolutionized heart care through natural means, now says the number one factor which determines how long we live is love and intimacy—even more than diet, drugs, or surgery![91]

As the last thirty years have demonstrated to millions of Americans, intimacy doesn't follow automatically from communication or nakedness or even sex. It's the mysterious element that can suddenly bloom between sexual partners and create an opening. A deepening. A beckoning. When it's there, the ground moves and the world seems clearer. Not surprisingly for so great a treasure, intimacy is not always easy to attain, or maintain. It takes the willingness and ability to do something that isn't always easy— fundamentally look beyond yourself and your own needs and desires.

The word intimacy can mean many things. It can signify closeness. Being involved sexually. Relating to our innermost self. The personal. The informal. And more. But our challenge here is to find out what the word really means for ourselves and our lovers. One thing's for sure: intimacy may be hard to define, but it's absolutely simple to recognize. It's a feeling, and a very good one too.

So let's look into this powerful urge for connection. This drive to know and be known is what separates men from mice, men from boys, and men from some of their own deepest fears. It also connects men in extraordinary ways to their own greatest potential, to their lovers, and no matter what their age, to the throbbing heartbeat of life itself in wonderful new ways.

FIVE PATHS TO INTIMACY

Get Real

From the perspective of evolution, intimacy is new. The ability to make distinctions between ourselves and others, and language itself, was acquired relatively recently.[92] That might explain why true intimacy is less common than many think. Sure, you can find literally tons of novels and movies and

CDs about love, but most of them offer romantic yearnings for love rather than the daily demands of intimacy. While intimacy begins in romance, its greatest rewards are realized over time.

Psychoanalyst Robert Johnson examines that distinction in an essay called "Stirring the Oatmeal."[93] The title refers to the kind of love that goes beyond romantic illusions—seeing our partner as she really is, and permitting her to see us that way too. It's in the "daily-ness" of life that we really get to know each other. Dealing with money, raising kids, cleaning the house—these are what bring us down from the clouds and land our feet on the floor.

But we needn't feel like we're wearing lead shoes. Johnson makes an interesting distinction between how we treat friends and lovers. In many ways, friends end up getting more respect. We often listen better to them, help, and respect them in ways we tend to lose sight of in long term love relationships. Johnson advocates making friends of our lovers.

This brings us to the psychological idea of projection. Some would say that romance is a matter of us turning our lovers into what we want and need them to be. Our initial passion is so intense because we're connecting to what we deeply need, instead of to who our lovers truly are. Because that can't be sustained through time, the magic fades and dissatisfaction settles in. Sooner or later our lover becomes a real person with her own needs; she can't and shouldn't always put ours first.

This is the great fork in the road. Will lovers become friends, or will they separate and look again for someone to project their needs onto and feel the intense rush of starting the cycle anew? Johnson chooses the former. Accept reality, he counsels. Appreciate your lover as she really is. Make friends with her.

Does that mean an end to sex and passion? Not when we begin to make love honestly. Illusions may fall away, but honest sex won't. We'll see why in the following section.

Be Intimate with Yourself

Thomas Moore, author of *Soul Mates*, looks at relationships through his lens of caring for the soul in everyday life. He notes that intimacy begins not in relationships, but within ourselves.[94] The lack of connection we feel with others may in fact be a lack of connection with parts of ourselves.

Some men feel guilty about just plain wanting to get away from it all. We like the deep emotional and physical satisfactions of intimacy, but at times feel the need to leave it all behind. The wise man, and woman, accepts this urge without conflict. Classic escapes like fishing, hiking, and making art have been joined by newer versions like hang-gliding and meditation.

It's just another side to the two-sided coin of union and independence. And while we all have plenty of occasion to wade knee-deep in social connections at work and/or home, many of us are spending less time face-to-face with solitude and ourselves. That's too bad, because solitude offers much-needed space for recharging our inner batteries and staying in touch with our innermost desires—and how they change.

We all learn very early in life that getting along in the world means suppressing personal urges. Of course that's realistic and helps our participation with family, peers, and community. But only by paying attention to our own desires, feelings, and attitudes do we know how to relate to those of others. Getting to know oneself and someone else are in fact the two sides to intimacy. When we're more open to our own strengths and weaknesses, we'll find more interest in those of our partners. Ditto for quirks, oddball notions, and irrational fears, yours and hers.

So whether you decide on an occasional weekend of hiking in the mountains or just a couple of hours lying on your back in the backyard, honor yourself. Keep in touch with what's stirring within. Maybe that boredom or restlessness is a sign that you need some time alone. Then come back and share your discoveries with those you love.

Being physically intimate with yourself brings the same benefits. Expanding your concept of masturbation is like expanding your concept of sex in general. Like learning to appreciate the full spectrum of lovemaking, instead of concentrating on your penis and orgasm, experience the sensitivity of other parts of your body. While some would label this as self-centered, it is in fact the basis of advanced sexual techniques (some leading to sex at its most spiritual) of Taoist and tantric sex—and it contributes much to the sex you share with your partner.

Be Yourself in Relationships

Some people use the word intimacy when referring to the satisfaction of getting what they need from someone else. That can certainly feel like intimacy, and may be part of it. But the only reliable source of intimacy is not what you receive, it's what you give. And being able to give comes from knowing and valuing oneself.

Needing someone else to make us feel good, while a natural impulse, can land us in hot water, especially in a long-term relationship, where the needs and aspirations of people change. David Schnarch, a psychologist who combines sex and marital counseling in a dynamic new way, makes a distinction between two basic types of intimacy: self-validated and other-validated.[95] In other words, while we may think we want intimacy, in fact what we're looking for from our partner is to make us feel accepted and good about ourselves. Real intimacy, he notes, doesn't always consist of cozy and happy times. It can sometimes feel intensely challenging. But in the process it can make us strong instead of weak, and re-ignite our sex lives as well.

The essence of this new message is that we all need to learn how to be ourselves, even when we feel pressure to be what someone else wants us to be. When two people do manage to be themselves (what Schnarch refers to as *differentiated*) and communicate their true preferences, the relationship can grow stronger, not weaker.

Sex, for example, gets more honest. More *intimate*. It sizzles, not because we're doing what's expected, but because we're tapping deep needs and the ability to give as good as we get. As Schnarch adds, this can fly in the face of traditional sex therapy and its reliance on sensate focus. When we dare to keep our eyes open during sex—literally and figuratively—we avoid the false spirals of manipulation, self-preservation, and fears of performance. Instead, we can enjoy love-infused wilds of mature sexuality.

Broaden Your Search for Intimacy

Many men yearn to lose themselves in an intimate relationship, yet at the same time insist on their independence. Psychologists relate this to their earliest experience with their mothers. As infants, boys need a mother's comfort, yet need to assert their own independence as well. It's a conflict most take with them throughout their lives, especially in their relationships with women.

Yes, intimacy can be deeply comforting. And healthy too. Studies confirm that men who have close confidants fare better than those without them in avoiding and recovering from serious illnesses ranging from heart disease to cancer to respiratory infections.[96] The lesson is clear: intimacy is good for your health.

But while we know intimacy feels good, and is good for us, there's something to be said for not expecting one person to satisfy all our needs for it. Although a long term relationship provides a safe haven from the stormy seas of life, some would argue that a deeper security includes friends and interests outside a primary relationship.

In this enlarged model of intimacy, a relationship consists of individuals growing stronger through their union. Jealousy won't be a problem because each partner wants the other to grow. Their relationship is not a world unto itself, but part of a larger community and world.

Of course this is not easy. It's easier to settle into the comfort of even a stale intimacy than to take risks and grow in an evolving connection with the world. Staying fresh requires some degree of experimentation. This needn't threaten a monogamous relationship. In fact it can nourish it. Sex, for instance, is more likely to remain a strong and nourishing part of a relationship not bound in habits. Sexual boredom can therefore be seen not as the inevitable destination of relationship, but merely signaling the need for more growth—for the relationship, and for you.[97]

Trust Intimacy

One of the biggest challenges with intimacy is trusting it. After all, you're opening yourself up, revealing your tender emotional underbelly. In other words, you're vulnerable, a state not many men feel comfortable with—especially after being taken advantage of once or twice.

Naturally, fear enters into the picture, and pain too. But that's when intimacy shines brightest. As John Welwood notes in *Challenges of the Heart*, intimate relationships have the power to heal emotional wounds if we let them.[98] He notes an emotional current in us that's equivalent to the Chinese idea of circulating bioenergy. And when in an intimate relationship we allow ourselves to feel and reveal parts of our heart that we've sealed off, we can safely blast through the protective walls and reach our ever-fresh hearts within. The mystery of that process is intimacy's gold. Of course we have to be sure that our partners are also willing to participate in the process. Reciprocity is the backbone of intimacy.

The safety of intimacy also allows us to explore the masculine in her and the feminine in us. Sure, some men like to make fun of that idea, but only those who don't understand its power. Typically men approaching middle age are more liable to consider it, men who have seen the futility of unrelenting machismo, hidden emotions, and superficial communication. They sense a wholeness that beckons. Whole new fields of possibility. Sexual and otherwise. Intimacy demands, and rewards. It always involves some risk. That's what being fully alive moment to moment entails. When you reach the point of wanting to be fully awake, and stop the lazy drift of risking nothing, you're ready.

When you're committed to intimacy, you're ready to leave the sexual minor leagues behind and ready to start making love in the majors.

KAMA SUTRA

It begins...

...on a Saturday night. A friend's parents are out of town and you're slow-dancing at a party in his basement. You can't believe how thrilling it is, arms around a girl, feeling her hair on your face. Someone has turned the lights low and a pulsing love song blares from a radio in the corner. The music ends. The two of you embrace for a long moment. For the first time ever, you smell a girl's smell. Then, staring into her eyes, you're vaguely aware of wood-paneling behind her, so you move her back two steps to the wall and press against her with your whole body and kiss her and she presses back where she means it, igniting a totally new feeling within you. A warmth. An energy. Suddenly the lights go on and you move away, slightly shocked and not realizing the magnitude of what just happened: you discovered sex. A very simple form, yes, but part of you just stepped out of childhood.

What's your next move? What you're feeling wasn't covered in Mr. Murphy's sex ed class in school. Where do you turn for answers when you're not even clear about the questions? For many of us, the information dribbled in slowly over a period of years.

Imagine being clear about sex from the get-go.

Sex would be a source of pleasure and power and fulfillment from youth forward, no matter how simple or complex the circumstance. You'd even have an idea of when to start.

But consider how you *really* learned about sex and how many detours you have endured since that first embrace: guilty visits in forbidden magazines, distorted sexual bragging on playgrounds, inappropriate groping, esteem-deflating rejections. Good sex education can make all the difference. And the best sex manual the world has ever seen is in the *Kama Sutra*.

In our time, Masters and Johnson's *Human Sexual Response* broke new ground. But valuable though it was, the reader had to wade through descriptions like "retrogression changes in the resolution phase." Whoa! Who wouldn't rather spend an adventurous evening in an erotic Indian garden?

LEARN FROM A MASTER

Over two thousand years ago in India, a man named Vatsyayana condensed ancient guides to love and sex in a master document called the *Kama Sutra*. The world of sex would never be quite the same.

The book's modern reputation stems from its specifics on sexual technique, which it delivers in detail. But most of those tips occur in one section, and the book contains seven in all. Vatsyayana puts sex within the whole of a man's life—social, cultural, economic, and spiritual. However much we'd like to think otherwise, some things haven't changed. Love and sex are never free. More than just desire and groans, sex calls for responsibility and balance in one's life.

True, the *Kama Sutra* is a mixed bag. Some of its suggestions are laughable by today's standards, such as applying ground camel bones to your eyelashes. Other examples would be received coolly in some quarters: a wife is advised not to visit her own family when her husband is traveling. But such peculiarities of a faraway time and culture are overshadowed by the wealth of sophisticated, creative—and useful—advice about love and sex.

Where else can you find a guide for integrating sex and money and spiritual considerations, or a sex manual that describes an astonishing variety of positions for intercourse? How about advice for kissing, foreplay, afterplay, oral sex, anal sex, masturbation, agonizingly gentle sex, surprisingly rough sex, group sex, sex toys, sex with prostitutes, sex in water, sexual preferences by geographical region, fantasies, massage oils, aphrodisiacs, advice on what kind of girl to date, when divorce is appropriate, when to sleep with a neighbor's wife, when to bite, scratch, and slap your lover, and when not to?

When it comes to sex, old Vatsyayana wrote the book!

LESSONS FROM *THE* BOOK OF LOVE

The *Kama Sutra* portrays the values and ways of an upper class gentleman and his society in a distant place and time. In some ways, the best approach to this book is anthropological. But it's not hard to separate the information that's merely interesting from what's applicable to your life tonight. Few of us need advice on whether to dally with a shepherd girl. But tweak the details and that advice is suddenly relevant to office politics. An anthropologist observes, but always with an eye to how those observations might

Kama Sutra, **The Movie**

In 1997, director Mira Nair's controversial film *Kama Sutra* was released to mixed reviews. Viewers looking mainly for steamy sex scenes found them, but the movie is not soft pornography in search of a plot. In fact, the student of *Kama Sutra,* the book, will find much of interest in this film.

The story follows a woman on her path from servant girl through her tribulations as a courtesan to her later enlightened realization of the meaning of her life. Viewers are transported to a 16th century India brought alive with sumptuous costumes and sets. There we see the intertwining destinies of a king, a queen, a sculptor, and Tara, the servant girl turned Kama Sutra practitioner, who, it must be said, ignites the film with eroticism.

In terms of the ancient text itself, the film bears an important message. Sex purely for the sake of pleasure or ego or power can't match the profound depth of sex in the full context of one's potential as a human being. That message is no less relevant today as we pivot into yet another millennium of human achievement and folly and sexual adventure.

enrich his own culture. The *Kama Sutra* offers much that can enrich your experience of sex.

Be Willing to Learn

One unfortunate, and widespread, illusion is that a man should arrive in manhood already a sexual master. And more, he should translate this innate knowledge into action whenever and wherever he's called upon to do so.

The *Kama Sutra* counsels otherwise. One has to be open, willing to learn, and ready to practice. Vatsyayana stresses the virtue of being in touch with your lover's state, of doing what's appropriate to her interest and response. He provides a wealth of techniques, but it's up to you to learn when and how they are best introduced. And that takes practice.

In this, he is very modern. He values a woman, her sensitivity, and her intelligence. Sure, if he were alive in America today, he might choose not to suggest she go to sleep after him and wake up earlier in order to best serve him. But what modern woman doesn't appreciate the lavish attention he suggests she receive?

Learn the Details

Where is the man who knows everything about sex? Some would claim the distinction, but only bores and liars, those for whom the Zen master would pour a cup of tea until overflowing, to illustrate how a man can't learn anything new when he is already full of himself.

The *Kama Sutra* is based in philosophy, but filled with details, a vast range of sexual possibilities to complete or complement a man's—or woman's—natural inclinations.

Feeling too gentle? Read the section on slapping and biting.

Been accused of being too rough? Read the advice on how to relax the virgin bride.

Ready for something new? Try one of the advanced, yoga-like positions for intercourse. The spin, for instance, where you begin in back of her and wind up in front, without having separated in the process.

The book addresses larger issues, and it focuses on details. Read it yourself and enjoy the discoveries.

KEGELS

The King Of All Sexercise

Elsewhere in this book you'll find physical exercises for stamina and flexibility (see the Exercise chapter). In this chapter you'll find exercises for sexual *gold*.

Kegel exercises are the key to optimum sex. No matter what your sexual goals, these exercises will help you reach them. From more confidence in the bedroom to multiple orgasms, Kegels are the royal route. No other exercises so specifically boost sexual health and fitness.

And most amazingly, they're easy to learn and you can do them anywhere and anytime, even while standing on line at the bank.

KEGEL BASICS

Kegel exercises are variations of one basic move: flexing and relaxing your love muscle. No, not *that* love muscle (there aren't any muscles in your penis). This love muscle is an informal name for the pubococcygeus (PC) muscle, also called the pelvic floor muscle.

The pelvis is the graceful set of bones connecting your spine with your legs. It has two sides (hip bones), a back (sacrum), and an open bottom and front. The PC muscle is the group of muscles spanning that open bottom, forming a floor of musculature with holes for the anus and base of the penis.

There's an easy way to find this muscle: feel it. Next time you urinate, stop the flow in midstream. You just flexed your PC muscle. You've also just done a Kegel exercise.

> **Kegels: Exercising for Sexual Gold**
>
> Are Kegel Exercises for you? They are if you're interested in:
> - greater ejaculatory control
> - more intense orgasms
> - multiple orgasms
> - boosting prostate health
> - raising your partner's satisfaction
> - maintaining passion in long-term relationships

DR. KEGEL TO THE RESCUE

The exercise's name comes from a gynecologist in California named Arnold Kegel, who had a wonderful idea. Some of his patients who had just given birth were dribbling urine upon coughing or even laughing. That was due to the extreme stretching their PC muscle had sustained while giving birth. Dr. Kegel suggested exercising the PC muscle to re-tone it, thus restoring continence. What he didn't know was that his exercise would improve their sex lives. They reported a major upgrade in their sexual pleasure. And when a woman flexes her toned PC muscle during sex, it means more pressure on the penis and...well, we know what that means.

THE JOY OF FLEXING

Dr. Kegel's discovery led to an awareness in the West of what has long been known in the Orient: an intimate connection between the PC muscles, the penis, and astonishing orgasms. For a man, strengthening the PC muscle takes sex to whole new levels of pleasure—for him and his partner.

When the PC muscle is flexed, it rises and exerts pressure on the prostate gland. A generally unrealized fact about the prostate gland is its role in orgasm.

The first stage of orgasm, noted by Masters and Johnson in their pioneering sex research in St. Louis, is called emission: the prostate releases its fluids which mix with sperm, a process men experience as an awareness of inevitability of orgasm. This point itself is called orgasm in the Oriental view, a separate event from ejaculation.

That's the crux—separating orgasm from ejaculation. In other words, it's possible to experience the pleasure of orgasm without the release of semen or loss of erection. In the West, that's revolutionary. In the Orient, it's lengthy, sexual bliss as usual. It's control over ejaculation. Intense orgasms. Multiple Orgasms. More about those in *Orgasms* and *Tantric Sex*. For now, let's get to the king of all sexercise.

JUST DO THEM

Few exercises are as simple, or powerful, as Kegels. Here are the basics:

PC Muscle Awareness

The first step is to experience the PC muscles directly. You can do that, as we've already seen, by using them to stop urination. Another way to feel them is to touch the area between the testicles and anus during ejaculation. The rhythmic pulsations you feel are contractions of the PC muscle.

When you first experiment, you might confuse your PC with your gluteus maximus (or butt) muscles. That's natural. Just keep simulating the act of stopping the flow of urine, and you'll get it.

PC Muscle Flexing

Now you're into real Kegels. Once you can flex the PC muscle at will, do it regularly. At first just flex and relax. Later flex and hold for three seconds. Then relax. Do only a few at first. Then do as many sets as feels right. Ten, twenty, or fifty or more throughout the day. Experiment and find what works best for you. What's important is doing them regularly, just as you would to benefit from any exercise.

You'll find that the opportunities for doing Kegels are endless. Do them while sitting at your desk, or waiting on line for food. Whatever. Hey, it feels good to use these mundane moments to pump up your love life.

The PC Muscle in Sex

Flexing the PC muscle during sex is where the fun really begins. After you've developed love muscle awareness and control, you'll have more awareness of, and control over, your orgasms. For starters, that means more control over when you ejaculate, which will please your partner. When you are able to clearly feel the pre-orgasm "orgasm" in the prostate, and slow to avoid ejaculation, you're on the road to multiple orgasms. More about the PC muscle, energy flow, and advanced techniques of multiple orgasms is in the *Taoist Sex* and *Tantric Sex* chapters. Those no-longer-secret practices involve partners using the energies of sex together in new and profound ways. They lead to the spiritual side of sex and high levels of health and longevity. And they begin with Kegel exercises.

KISSING

For some men, kissing barely registers on the pleasure meter. Seems a shame, because they're ignoring a potent path to intimacy and ardor. And they're probably ignoring one of their lover's major hot spots.

Other men have long made kisses a priority. They understand the pleasure and power involved. And they know that in giving great kisses they simultaneously receive them.

Peak sexual fitness demands a comfort with kissing. For a great lover, kisses encourage confidence and connection. That's why for him a great kiss is always prime time news.

HOW TO KISS YOUR WAY TO PASSION

What exactly *is* a kiss, anyway? Not much more than a squirrel call until you touch another person. Then it becomes a subtle invitation, a firm promise, and kindling for passion, among other things. Let's explore the ability and readiness to kiss for romance, love, and passion.

Here, as elsewhere in our journey, we're creating categories for the purpose of discussion. Variations abound, obviously, and using them is the mark of an amorous master. But let's look at the kisses that broadly correspond to three stages of relationship, whether for a night or a lifetime:

Romance/Lip Kissing

You're beyond the cheek kisses of friendship. You've arrived at romance, and serious kissing is a giveaway sign of serious emotional chemistry. It starts with the lips. Lips are sensitive areas, sensitive enough to send some women all the way to orgasm. So make an art of these kisses.

Memories of first kisses can last forever, so make them count. Over a special meal, in the rain, on the beach—the setting can help, but what's important is the kiss itself. Sheer voltage is less important than a new connection, a circular flow of interest. Try some delicacy, ya big lug!

Love/Tongue Kissing

The relationship has progressed, and so has the kissing. For some, it's naturally time for tongue (or French) kissing. Now the tongue is involved with more than whispering sweet nothings. The penetration of your lover's mouth suggests delights to come, and often accompanies them too. The key here is timing. Loose your tongue when your lover is ready and willing to receive it. Not before. How to know? Experimentation. Practice. Dedication. Just like golf, right? Well, only if you're really passionate about your five iron.

Passion/Body Kissing

Now the action is hot and heavy. Doesn't matter if you're on the picnic blanket, in the rear of a van, or back in the bedroom. It's exploration time. New worlds beckon. Shoulders, breasts, stomachs, thighs, feet—wherever your, and her, preferences lie. For some, the destination tends to be right between her legs. More on this under *Oral Sex*. Suffice it to say that whether you're on a passionate train to Union Station, or just motoring along the byways of noncoital sex, body kissing is a sure route to deep intimacy and pleasure.

Nine Indispensable Kissing Tips

One man's rule is another's exception—too many impulses motivate kissing for absolute generalizations to apply. Nonetheless, the following basics offer a sound foundation on which to improvise your unique approach.

1. *Make sure your mouth is fit to kiss*

   Cleanliness is the key. Fresh breath and smooth skin are good, but there are many bearded smokers with satisfied lovers. There's a difference between the scent of tobacco and halitosis. Dental floss and regular brushing are important. Keep breath mints handy, or, to impress the Earth Mother type, suck a clove or munch a sprig of parsley.

2. *Make sure your kisses are wanted*

   This applies from the simplest of kisses to the most passionate. Knowing when your kisses are welcome can be tricky. You might have to kiss to know for sure, which works when she's looking for an assertive note. Or if the moment allows, simply ask. But don't be afraid to surprise her with a kiss. A surprise kiss has a power all its own, especially when planted in a surprising place or at a surprising time— when she didn't know you were behind her, or in public, or when she's still sleeping.

   However, the more intense your unwanted kisses, the more negative her reaction. If your face is stinging from a sharp slap, you can reasonably conclude your kiss was unwanted. And remember, a lovebite, or hickey, is in fact a bruise, so be damn sure she wants one before bestowing it.

Overall, remember that a kiss is a mutual act, and highly individual. Try a variety of kisses and find out which works for her, and you. Find the balance that works for the moment at hand.

3. *Approach each kiss as an exploration*

   There are far too many possibilities in kissing to allow its magic to fade. Keep it fresh—even in long relationships. Kisses mix well with nibbling, licking, blowing, and sucking. Put on your explorer's cap and sail into whatever territory arises. The pleasures are all the more intense for being uncharted.

4. *Vary your kisses*

   Short and long, wet and dry, hard and soft, quiet and noisy, lips and ears—variety is the spice of kisses. Mix your assertiveness and receptivity too. Like the tango, kissing takes two. Unlike the tango, however, there are no rules, only an end: connection and pleasure.

5. *Make good grooming a priority*

   First impressions condition first kisses. Your hair and dress figure heavily into first, and subsequent, impressions. Just as kissing is often the first stage of lovemaking, grooming is the first stage in kissing. The key is looking at yourself from her point of view (a worthy talent to cultivate in many areas of sexuality and relationship). Does she want to be close to your face? Are you attracting her? Good questions to ponder.

6. *Don't underestimate the power of kissing*

   If you tend to think of kissing only as foreplay, try making it the focus of your next lovemaking. Linger. Savor. Emotional rewards will multiply. Paradoxically, however, don't be surprised if your focused attention brings forth a high tide of passion and accompanying physical rewards.

7. *Don't hurry kissing*

   Sure, there's a time and a place for a quickie. But as a rule, the enlightened lover knows that the intensity of arousal directly relates to the intensity and pleasure of orgasm.[99] And taking your time with kissing is one of the best ways to build big arousal.

8. *Enjoy the sound of kissing*

   Don't be embarrassed by the smacks and other sounds of kissing. Enjoy them! Again, it's a mutual thing. But if she likes it, enjoy these sounds as much as all other sounds of lovemaking.

9. *Try the kissing game*

   Although one lover wins, the other doesn't exactly lose since the goal is to excite both. Begin with a good solid kiss, and then each lover tries to take the other's lips into his or her mouth as described in the *Kama Sutra*.[100] The game can progress, by surprise or otherwise, into an effort to capture both of your lover's lips at once, or to combat of tongues. Where will it lead? Perhaps to laughter, perhaps to passion.

USE THE LEGENDARY POWER OF KISSING

Imagine you're a frog. The world sure looks different from a lily pad, yes? Wait—here comes the most beautiful woman you've ever seen. Now she's bending over, kissing you, and POOF! you're a prince living happily ever after.

There are thousands of such stories from cultures around the world. It's noteworthy that they frequently involve a kiss. Kissing and transformation are intimately linked. It's about changing the mundane to magic, and indifference to passion. Kiss often and find out for yourself.

MASSAGE

Baffling but true: some men still snicker at the mention of massage. Why? How could something so powerfully healing—and potentially erotic—be so routinely dismissed? Must be the old male bugaboo of needing to appear tough and none too sensitive. If you still subscribe to that edition of yesterday's news, wake up and smell the rose oil! Take this quick tour of massage—what it is, what it offers you, and a few how-to basics. Then warm up those hands, pal, and prepare for the magic of giving, and receiving, a massage.

FULL-BODY BENEFITS FOR HEALTH AND SEX

The Ancient Egyptians used its curative power. So did the Greeks, Romans, and Chinese, among others. And now, thanks to the resurgence of natural healing, more and more American men are discovering the surprising power of massage to heal and rejuvenate their bodies, minds, and spirits.

If you think massage is about muscles, you're right, but only partially so. According to Elliot Greene, massage therapist and former president of the American Massage Therapy Association, massage can indeed prevent injury, speed healing, and tone muscles, but it also offers other circulation and nervous system benefits.[101]

A good massage boosts blood flow, encouraging a healthy supply of nutrients to cells all over the body (which, as we've seen, is good for a man's sexual response). It also encourages the removal of cellular waste by promoting the movement of lymph fluid, which depends on the movement of muscles to do its job.

The nervous system gets a helping hand as well. Massage can relax nerves with easy, flowing strokes, and/or energize them with more vigorous techniques. It tones the skin, keeping it in prime shape to do its important job as intermediary between our inner and outer life.

COMMUNICATE BY TOUCH

Today we're more productive at work, and with more labor-saving appliances and machines than ever before, more productive at home too. We pocket our wages and buy the things we need, and a few we don't. You can certainly make a case for life-is-good.

But we also work long hours, commute long distances, and zip around doing errands in what used to pass for free time. The general picture includes much to be thankful for—and much we'd prefer to ignore, like stress, jangled nerves, and less time for luxurious, satisfying sex. Massage can't solve all your problems, but it can help slow you

> ### An Important Caution
> Massage isn't always advisable.[102] The spread of an infectious disease, for example, can be encouraged by a massage. Also, some inflammations, injuries, and other medical or psychological conditions might be adversely affected. If you're in doubt about how this might apply to you or your partner, consult your doctor or a certified massage therapist.

down, banish stress, promote health, and provide a reliable bridge to deeply satisfying moments, sexual and otherwise.

It does so through the remarkable power of touch. In a complicated world, the here-and-now of massage encourages a strong connection with your partner. As we've seen, words are often necessary to relay important sexual information, but for some messages, words can't compare with the direct and immediate effect of warm hands stroking oiled skin.

For building intimacy, for communicating that you're involved and that you care, massage is a top-notch technique everyone can learn. Let's take a look at how it's done.

BACK TO THE PRESENT

The basic tool kit for massage couldn't be much simpler. All you really need is your hands. Massage oil will help, as will creating a calm atmosphere. Beyond that, it's all a matter of your desire to give, and receive, which brings up an interesting point right at the get-go. You can give a massage, and receive one, but the two aren't mutually exclusive. Breathing deeply, focusing on your partner, paying attention to *her* breathing and the state of her muscles and emotions, can create a profound meditative state. That in turn helps you focus better, and has its own rewards in terms of bringing you into the present, which is always a nourishing experience. So let's get back to the room you're in for this massage. We'll concentrate on sensual massage. Sure, there are all kinds of variations and levels of formality. Massage can turn into, or start as, foreplay. It can be mutual and simultaneous. But for now, she's naked with her eyes closed, waiting.

Make sure she's warm enough for comfort without clothes on or a top sheet. Whether or not you're naked is optional. Neutral, soft music and candles encourage a suitable atmosphere. The goal here (at least for the first part) is relaxation, and whatever contributes to that is a plus. Have enough padding beneath her for comfort and support if you're not in bed. Scented candles or incense? Depends on your massage oil. You can think of oil as lube for the job, or adding the sensuous, slippery essence of fragrant plants. It's her skin, which do you think she'd prefer?

THE POWER OF AROMATHERAPY

Essential oils are more popular than ever, and they're fueling the rising popularity of aromatherapy. You may have heard this word and figured it was some New Age hype about misting the air with perfume. Well, sort of. Actually, the word was coined by a French physician in the early part of this century to refer to the medicinal use of essential oils, which are distilled from the oil glands of certain plants. When diffused into air they do impart a variety of aromas, and each affects us differently as we breathe them in. Some soothe, some energize, some are reputed to help with headaches, heartburn, and many other ailments and conditions.

And those same oils are absorbed through the skin for a direct internal effect. So, yes, massage oils lubricate the skin and enable you to stroke and knead in ways not possible without them. But they also bring an organic power to the mix, and of course powerfully sensual aromas, which she will appreciate. And you will too.

You can buy various commercial blends of massage oil, or blend your own with a carrier oil from seeds (sunflower, soya, etc.) or nuts (such as walnut or almond). Try the essential oils of rose, ylang ylang, jasmine, sandalwood, or patchouli, or others. Most oils are too concentrated to apply without diluting them. Ask at a natural foods and/or herb store for more details. For now, let's get back to your partner, who has been waiting patiently for your tender hands.

RELAX AND SOOTHE HER

Okay, the atmosphere's perfect; you've rubbed a small amount of oil in your hands to warm it to skin temperature, and you're ready to begin. Where and how do you start? Needless to say, there's no rule book. Start wherever it

---

Hands and Fingers: tools of the trade

Your hands are incredibly versatile massage tools. Just think of all the different ways to use them: applying deep pressure with the heel, or base, of your hand; gentle tapping with finger pads or tips; chopping with the sides of your palms; probing deeply with thumbs; gentle slapping with full palm and fingers. And your finger joints allow your hands to mold perfectly to your partner's body as you glide them sensuously across the hills and valleys of her body. Hands are warm, expressive, and sensitive too, relaying messages about the state of the skin and muscles you're massaging. Remarkable!

---

feels right. Just as we saw in the *Exercise* chapter, it helps to think of the body as divided into several sections. Think neck, head, chest, back, arms, hands, abdomen, groin, thighs, lower legs, and feet. Where you start depends on your mood and respective intentions. We'll assume that relaxation will be your initial goal. So let's begin with her lying on her stomach, enabling you to start with long, soothing strokes up her back. But feel free to start wherever you want.

Get into a position where you can move freely and be secure enough for lifting her arm or head. Try kneeling either by her side or straddling her head. Use a flat-handed stroke with medium pressure from the small of her back slowly up on either side of the spine to her neck to the top of her shoulders.

If she's lying on her back to start, use the same long strokes from her abdomen up to her chest, then fan your hands out finishing on top of her shoulders. Repeat slowly.

Massage can incorporate lifting as well as stroking. Gently lifting her arms or head or legs offers a welcome release from the force of gravity, compounding the soothing nature of your effort.

Next, try a mix of strokes on her legs and arms. Vary the pressure and speed of your strokes. Knead larger muscles between your hands. Fan your hands as above, or stretch skin and muscles by moving your hands in opposite directions. Use your thumbs for smaller muscles like those at the base of the neck or calf muscles. These are the basic strokes of Swedish massage, and are used all over the body to relax and/or stimulate.

Other schools of massage such as Shiatzu and Reflexology are based on stimulating the meridians, or paths of energy flowing through the body, to release energy blocks which create soreness, pain, and disease. Whether or not you accept that explanation of muscle pain, for example, you might be

The Awesome Power of a Foot Rub

A foot rub is a surprisingly powerful massage. For a complex combination of bones and cartilage that carry a person's weight all day, feet are very sensitive. Again, start by warming the oil or lotion in your hands. Then use a combination of gliding strokes and pressures from heel to toe. Gently slap the heel. Rock your knuckles across the arch. Tap all over with firm finger tips. Use your fingers to gently twist and squeeze each toe. When finished, let her absorb the effects in silence. Listen to her feedback. If you're lucky, she'll reciprocate!

surprised to find how easy it is to locate them, and how welcome and effective your attention can be. Try thumb pressure on her upper back muscles, probing slightly deeper to feel for tense muscles; they feel tight and cordlike. Small circles and larger strokes with your thumb tips can help relieve the tension.

Whichever method you choose for these initial, relaxing strokes, expect an effect quickly. Her tension (and yours) begins to melt away, your connection is strong, and the intimacy is building. If you're both willing, through shared assumption or prior agreement, extend the massage into more intimate, erotic pleasures. Don't spring that intention out of nowhere, however; it could be most unwelcome. But if you're both interested, get ready to enter a garden of passionate delights.

BUILDING EROTIC ENERGY

Erotic massage may produce passion, but it follows common sense. Breasts, nipples, groins, and buttocks are hot spots. Tenderness is the keyword. Strategic kisses communicate caring.

There are surprises, though, and they vary between individuals. Rubbing ear lobes, inner thighs, toes, and even breasts can make some women swoon and leave others cold. You need to explore and find out what works.

She's relaxed. Your efforts so far have been appreciated. Now it's time to light an erotic fire. What matters most is that your attention and tender touch make her feel cared for and pampered. Arouse her by moving to one of her erogenous zones. Glide your hands around her breasts and hold them in your hands. Gently rub a nipple between your fingers. If she makes a gesture or sound of appreciation, obviously you're on the right track. When you're ready to move on, sit above her head, which you can gently lift and move, again giving her the sensation of floating free of gravity. Then gently move to her face, and rub or tap it lovingly, avoiding her eyes due to their sensitivity to touch. Or move to her legs, varying firm strokes or kneading with feather-light passes over her inner thighs.

SPREAD THE WEALTH

No, we're not talking about spreading legs. At least not yet. Rather, now that she's sexually aroused, try long strokes down and up her legs, or stomach and chest, or back; move that erotic energy through the rest of her body. Then maybe it's the perfect time for a bath, shower, hot tub, or dream-laden sleep. A glass of wine under the stars. Or continuing by her swelling, moistening, and receiving you into her, where you can continue the most full-bodied of massages. The possibilities are limited only by your imagination.

MASSAGE IN THE WORLD

Joseph has a good job in a marketing firm, a fat 401(k) plan, and a peach of a girlfriend. He thinks he should be sleeping better than he has been lately, but knows he feels uneasy about something Joan, his girlfriend, told him. She said she needs more from their sex than she's getting. More what? he asked. He could have predicted her answer: more touching.

It makes Joe nervous because his last girlfriend said the same thing before their relationship soured. His tendency is to hurry through foreplay to get to the main event, as his closest buddies call it. But now he likes the emotional connection he shares with Joan, and wants to do the right thing. A friend suggested reading about erotic massage, which he did, looking forward to trying some of the techniques.

The next time they were together, he asked Joan if she wanted a massage. Obviously surprised, and pleased, after a few moments she answered yes. He helped her take her clothes off and she lay down on the blankets and sheet he spread out in front of his fireplace. Then he proceeded to give her a thirty minute massage. Joan smiled or sighed through most of it, especially when he started lingering on her breasts. Joseph discovered that her toes and inner thighs were also particularly responsive.

He was surprised, and of course delighted, when she started touching him the way she did when she wanted sex. He rubbed some of the massage oil he had used on Joan over his thighs, stomach, and chest. Then he lay on top of her and slid slowly up and down and back and forth across her body for several minutes. He had never felt such physical pleasure outside of intercourse in his life. And when he was ready to enter her, she was ready too.

By the time they were done, she had tears in her eyes. They hugged and fell asleep in front of the fire, entwined in deep intimacy.

MASTURBATION

Whack off. Beat the dummy. Self-abuse. The names are bad news, and so are the alleged results: blindness, hairy palms, slumped shoulders. Since when has masturbation been such a problem? Well, at least since Genesis 38:9, when Onan sinned by spilling his seed on barren ground. Ever since, countless males have spilled their seed on a bed of guilt.

The Old Testament's judgment hasn't dimmed masturbation's attraction though. Twentieth century sex surveys (the only kind there are) differ on the number of men that masturbate, but a safe range is 30 to 80%. And one recent survey painted a surprising picture of who is masturbating and why: married people were much more likely to masturbate.[103] The survey's authors conclude that masturbation is more often part of an active sex life than a substitute for partnered-sex in a solo lifestyle.

So what is masturbation, and why all the hubbub? Traditional definitions vary, but the gist is *genital excitation, usually to orgasm, by means other than intercourse.* Sounds innocent enough. But don't tell that to Joyce Elders, the former Surgeon General, relieved of her job partly because she suggested masturbation deserves a place in sex education.

One of the foundations of this book is that sexual ignorance too often leads to sexual anxiety and sexual problems. Reversing that process moves back from problems and anxiety and ignorance to a fresh start and a new line to robust sexual fitness. That includes a new look at masturbation.

Anti-Masturbation Fever

In his book *American Sex Machines, The Hidden History of Sex at the U.S. Patent Office,* Hoag Levins presents some scary evidence of technology in service of sexual morality.[104] One device, patented in 1903, is an anti-masturbation harness: a strap worn around the waist with an attached tube, in which a penis was inserted. When an erection pushed a sensor in the tube, the device produced an electric shock and/or rang a bell. Gad zooks!

We're not here to debate the moral side of sex, solo or otherwise. We assume sex is a healthy part of human life, and suggest we should pay attention when something as common as masturbation has such a negative aura—especially when many sexologists are now presenting a more positive picture. The fact is, today it's easy to find reference to masturbation as innocent self-exploration, self-pleasuring, and other terms not formerly associated with the act. So let's take a look at this much-maligned aspect of sexuality, and see what it might hold for sexual health and fitness.

RELAX, ENJOY, AND LEARN

Self-pleasuring? Isn't that too self-centered for a mature adult? Absolutely not! As David Schnarch points out in his book *Passionate Couples,* there's a crucial difference between self-centered and self-centering, and the latter plays an important part in strengthening a relationship, the individuals in it, and the sex they have together.

There's nothing trivial about learning your sexual preferences, enjoying them, and communicating them to others. Much of today's most forward-looking sexual theory starts with the importance of knowing what turns you on. Hands-on learning—and relearning—is where it starts. There's no better way to cleanse the confusing layers of should's and should-not's that we all gathered while growing up.

And more: self-knowledge can form a foundation for new levels of sexual satisfaction for you and your lover, such as deeper and multiple orgasms for both. Ultimately, it starts with learning, or relearning, to feel your penis—and your testicles, perineum, prostate, and PC muscle.

Obviously, there are no rules in masturbation. But there's a lot more to it than an adolescent under sheets with a skin mag. In fact, that image might be a good place to start. Who's to say that those first stirrings of sexuality, when hidden and guilt-ridden and rushed, are the origins of not only many men's attitudes about sex, but of problems too, like premature ejaculation? By the way, this discussion assumes you don't have health conditions that might be adversely affected by the suggestions made. Consult with your doctor before starting any new health or fitness exercises, the following included.

Give yourself permission to relax, feel, and learn. As we let the old model of masturbation go, a new one appears in its place. It's you finding new sexual awareness, power, and pleasure.

EIGHT TIPS FOR THE NEW MASTURBATION

The New Masturbation? That's right, it's a new twist on an old standby. Masturbation isn't a race, it's not necessarily about photos of naked women (although there's no reason to exclude them), and there's no need for embarrassment. Of course, any male who has ever masturbated has arrived at his own preferences. But here are a few suggestions to enhance the experience.

Think of it as self-pleasuring or whatever allows you to do it freshly. There's no reason for speeding to orgasm. There's no reason to hide your feelings, and there are plenty of reasons for feeling the sensations. Yes, it's a private act, yet it doesn't have to be done alone. Here, then, are eight tips to practice the new masturbation for fun, pleasure, and knowledge.

1. *Relax*

   Set aside some uninterrupted time. Get comfortable. If you're feeling tense, take some time to unwind. Exercising, stretching, or a bath beforehand can help. If you know how to meditate, that can help establish a sense of presence, which is important. No one is telling you what to do or what to feel. You're exploring that for yourself. And establishing a clear, relaxed state of mind and body is the best way to proceed.

2. *Start with your body*

   Lie down wherever feels comfortable. There's no need to grab your penis right off the bat. Think of sex as a whole body thing. Rub your hands together and place them over your closed eyes. Enjoy their warmth. Place a hand over your chest and feel it rise and fall as you breathe. As you relax, feel your breathing move from your upper chest deeper to your lower chest and abdomen. Place a hand on your belly and feel it rise and fall. Gently rub your thighs. Whatever.

3. *Touch*

   One of the hallmarks of this practice is a new state of presence. You want to be present for the act. If you like to use photos to arouse yourself, feel free. But at some point come back to the sensations your touch evokes. You're exploring, so be present for incoming news from your fingertips.

4. *Lubricate*

   Some touching feels right with dry hands, some feels better with lubrication. Lotions feel and smell good. Body powder too. Or massage oils, which last longer than lotion. Experiment. Find which feels best for you and each kind of touch.

5. *Explore your penis*

   OK, so it sounds strange. Why not just shake hands with an old friend, right? Well, think of it as a new friend, one you're meeting for the first time. Feel its whole length. Gently squeeze. Notice where it's most sensitive. Then start slowly stroking. Notice how the sensations get stronger. And feel better. If you're used to fast stroking only, slow it down. (In fact, if you're noticing that your penis seems less sensitive than it used to, try only slow stroking for awhile and see if that makes a difference.)

6. *Explore your other genitals*

    Here's a big payoff. Being open to what's happening leads to much more than orgasm as usual, or even health and sexual fitness as usual. Read on.

    Feel your testicles. Cup them. Visualize them strong and healthy. Some therapists suggest pulling down on them to slow a too-quickly approaching orgasm. Acquaint yourself with your perineum, the area between your testicles and your anus. You can feel your PC muscle here (more about that in *Kegels*), and the base of your penis extending back to your pubic bone.

7. *Explore orgasm*

    As you'll read in the chapters *Taoist Sex* and *Ejaculation,* there's more to orgasm than ejaculation. Masturbation is a good place to learn the difference. What some call a prostate orgasm occurs when that gland releases its fluid to mix with semen. Ejaculation occurs when the PC muscle contracts, forcing the semen up and out of the penis. Approach orgasm and stop. Feel what's going on, and where. Besides helping to prolong and deepen your experience of intercourse, this is the threshold to more advanced sexual techniques discussed in the chapters on *Tantric* and *Taoist sex.* If or when orgasm comes, enjoy it without reservation. Shake, rattle, and roll. Twist and shout!

8. *Do it with someone else*

    Shared masturbation takes the above material to another level. For learning more about what excites your lover, for safe peace-of-mind sex, or just for a change of pace, shared masturbation is great stuff! And if you feel pressure about performing, here's how to retrace your steps back to enjoyment. Don't exclude playfulness. Use words and touch for sharing questions and discoveries. Many of the techniques described above apply here. In many cases, more so. Like the initial relaxation phase, which can be expanded into sensuous massage, complete with essential oils and exotic aromas. Like the whole body aspect, which makes for great foreplay. Again, there's no need to rush to orgasm. In fact, experiment with not pursuing orgasm; instead concentrate on the symphony of sensations and pleasure as you give, receive, and enjoy languid and/or torrid sex without intercourse. Many men find masturbation with a lover present quite intense.

MEDICATIONS

Medical drugs are so commonly prescribed and consumed today that few people concern themselves with unwanted side effects. Unless the Federal Drug Administration pulls a drug from pharmacy shelves, most people don't research potential problems every time their doctor gives them a prescription (even though extensive reference material on the subject is available at the local library).

But once you've personally experienced one of those side effects, the subject suddenly becomes relevant. For thousands of men, that happens when a side effect impacts their sexuality, in the form of reduced sexual desire, erectile dysfunction (ED), or problems with ejaculation, their testicles, Peyronie's disease, or priapism.

While the FDA's rigorous testing process is designed to minimize unforeseen dangers, not all problems are avoided. In fact the government's General Accounting Office recognizes that 51% of pharmaceutical drugs approved by the FDA eventually cause significant side effects not discovered before their approval.[105]

A FAMOUS CASE IN POINT

Viagra is a notable example of surprise side effects. Although happily taken to correct erectile dysfunction by millions of men—many of whom don't mind minor side effects like headache, upset stomach, or blue-tinged vision—over a hundred have died from heart attacks linked to the drug. The FDA and the drug's manufacturer have added warnings to the drug's packaging regarding men with previous histories of heart problems (a group not studied before the drug's approval). Also added to the labels were cautions about rare incidences of prolonged and dangerous erections lasting more than four hours.

ASK, DON'T ASSUME

Because of the vast number of variables in testing, that some side effects only appear after a drug has been on the market awhile shouldn't surprise us. The same is true in each man's individual experience; sometimes a sexual side effect may not appear until he's taken the drug for many months. And further complication is that a sexual problem may result from the disease or condition itself, not its treatment.

Doctors are busy. Given their workload, it's understandable that they may not know every side effect of every drug. And many other side effects are considered more serious than sexual problems. So if you suspect that a sexual problem is linked to medications you're taking, assume your share of responsibility for finding out for sure.

First of all, ask your doctor. He may be aware of side effects or he may not. But, most likely, he will be able substitute another drug. Also, depending on your condition and medication, he may try reducing the dose or, in some cases, suggest a "vacation" from the drug for short periods, as is sometimes done successfully with antidepressants.

But please note: Ask your doctor about making any change in drug type, dosage, or frequency of administration—never adjust them on your own. Doing so could seriously endanger your health.

If you're embarrassed about asking your doctor about this subject, ask anyway. It's too important to ignore. And if he doesn't give you a satisfying answer, find another doctor or clinic for someone more receptive to your problem. You might also want to consider a natural remedy or therapy. Many books and magazines in that field are available in your local library or natural foods store.

MEDICAL DRUGS AND SEXUAL SIDE EFFECTS

The following pages list drugs that have been associated with sexual side effects. Though surprisingly long, it is by no means complete. New drugs—and new side effects—regularly appear.

Men shouldn't worry about sexual side effects if not having sexual problems. But when those problems do occur, the role of drugs should be considered. A simple change of medication may provide welcome relief.

Be aware that the study of sexual side effects does not receive the intensive attention or rigid controls as other research does. Therefore your own experience and input from your doctor are the best guide of all.

The columns on the next pages list *drug type* (generic name) alphabetically, *brand name(s)*, and conditions for which they're prescribed (note: many drugs are prescribed for more than one medical condition). Not all brand names are listed for each drug. Dosage may be a factor in a drug's potential for side effects.

Consult your doctor or pharmacist for more detailed information.

DRUGS LINKED TO NEGATIVE MALE SEXUAL SIDE EFFECTS

Drug Type	Brand Name(s)	Side Effects*
Acute mental disorder medications:		
chlorpromazine	Ormazine, Thorazine	DES, EJAC, PRI
fluphenazine	Modecate, Permitril	ED
haloperidol	Haldol, Peridol	DES, ED, EJAC, PRI
lithium	Carbolith, Eskalith, Lithotabs	ED
mesoridazine besylate	Serentil	DES, ED
molindone	Moban	DES, EJAC
prochlorperazine	Compazine, Stemetil, Pro-Iso	ED
promazine	Sparine	ED
trifluoperazine	Stelazine, Suprazine	EJAC, PRI
Alcohol-abuse medication:		
disulfiram	Antabuse, Cronetal	DES, ED
Anxiety medications:		
chlordiazepoxide	Librax, Librium, Lipoxide	DES, ED
clorazepate	Tranxene	DES,ED
diazepam	Intensol, Meval, Valium	DES, ED
meprobamate	Milprem, Meditran, Tranmep	ED
oxazepam	Serax	ED
trifluroperazine	Solazine, Stelazine, Suprazine	ED, EJAC
Cancer medications:		
busulfan	Myleran	DES, ED
chlorambucil	Leukeran	DES, ED
cytarabine	Arabino-sylcytosine, Cytosar	DES
melphalan	L-PAM, Alkeran	DES, ED
procarbazine	Ibenzmethyzin, Matulane	DES, ED
vinblastine sulfate	Velban, Velsar	DES, ED
vincristine sulfate	LCR, Oncovin, Vincasar PFS	DES

Side Effects: DES = reduced desire, ED = Erectile dysfunction, EJAC = ejaculation problem, FERT = reduced fertility, PRI = Priapism

Drug Type	Brand Name(s)	Side Effects*
Cardiovascular medications:		
chlorthalidone	Combipres, Demi-regroton, Hygroton, Uridon	ED
chlorothiazide	Aldoclor, Azide, Diuril	ED
clofibrate	Atromid-S	ED
clonidine	Catapres, Combipres	DES, ED, EJAC
digitalis	Ouabain	ED
disopyramide	Napamide, Norpace, Rythmodan	ED
guanethidine	Ismelin, Esimil	ED, EJAC, PRI
hydrochlorothiazide	Aldactazide, Aldoril, Esidrix, Micrin, Timolide, Zide	ED
methylodopa	Aldomet	DES, EJAC
metoprolol	Betaloc, Lopressor	ED
pargyline	Eutonyl	ED
phenoxybenzamine	Dibenzyline	ED, EJAC
phentolamine	Regitine	ED
prazosin	Furazosin, Minipress	DES, ED, PRI
propranolol	Inderal, Ipran, Intensol	ED
reserpine	HHR, Hydroprin, Serpate	DES, ED, EJAC
spironolactone	Alatone, Aldactone, Sironazole, Sincomen	ED
Depression medication:		
amitriptyline	amitril, elavil, emitrip, endep, etrafon, levate, triavil	DES, ED
amoxapine	Asendin	DES, EJAC
chlorpromazine	Chlorpromanyl, Largactil, Promapar, Thorazine	ED, PRI
clomipramine	Anafranil	ED, EFAC
desipramine	Norpramin, Pertofrane	DES, ED
doxepin	Adapin, Sinequan	DES
fluoxetine hydrochloride	Prozac	ED
imipramine	Hanimine, Impril, Janimine, Tipramine, Tofranil	DES, ED

Side Effects: DES = reduced desire, ED = Erectile dysfunction, EJAC = ejaculation problem, FERT = reduced fertility, PRI = Priapism

Drug Type	Brand Name(s)	Side Effects*
isocarboxazide	Marplan	ED
maprotiline	Ludiomil	DES, ED
nortriptyline	Aventyl, Pamelor	DES, ED
phenelzine	Nardil	ED
protriptyline	Triptil, Vivactil	DES, ED
thioridazine	Mellaril, Novoridazine	ED, EJAC, PRI
trazodone	Desyrel, Trialodine	DES, ED, PRI
tripramine maleate	Surmontil	DES, ED
traxodone hydrochloride	Desyrel, Trialodine	ED

Gastrointestinal medications:

atropine	Atropisol, Bellergal, Kinesed, Donnatal, Logen, Uretron	ED
cimetidine	Peptol, Tagamet	DES, ED, FERT
metoclopramide	Emex, Maxeran, Reglan	DES, ED, FERT
propantheline	Norpanth, ProBanthine	ED
ranitidine	Zantac	DES, ED
sulfasalazine	azulfidine, S.A.S.-Enteric	FERT

Parkinson's Disesase medications:

biperidin	Akineton	ED
cycrimine	Pagitane	ED
levodopa	Dopar, Parda, Sinemet	DES, EJAC, PRI
trihexyphenidyl	Artane	ED
procyclidine	Kemadrin	ED

Prostate Medications:

estradiol	Ertrogel, Estrace, Dioval,Genora, Menaval, Nordette	DES, ED, EJAC
finasteride	Proscar	DES, ED
flutamide	Eulexin	DES, ED
goserelin	Zoladex	ED
leuprolide	Leuprorelin, Lupron	DES, ED

Side Effects: DES = reduced desire, ED = Erectile dysfunction, EJAC = ejaculation problem, FERT = reduced fertility, PRI = Priapism

MIDLIFE AND SEX

In 1930, Dr. Carl Jung wrote an astonishing essay about you.

He called it *The Stages of Life*. In it, the Swiss psychiatrist noted how a man's life can be divided into three parts: a first half, a second half, and a transition time between them called middle life.[106]

But there's more: he saw youth and early adulthood not as a peak period of never-to-be-equaled vitality and happiness, but as behavior and accomplishments often driven by the expectations of parents, wife, or peers.

Middle life, in his view, is a period of adjustment, of realizing one's true self and calling.

Then the second half of life becomes the creative and truly passionate part. Sexually and otherwise, intimacy comes easier, achievements are more meaningful, and true fulfillment more probable—if one successfully navigates the straits of midlife.

Dr. Jung therefore suggested you consider midlife upheavals like divorce or job loss not as random suffering or unjust fate. Rather, they form a period of *transition*. If midlife is a riddle, growth and transformation are the answer. Nowhere is this truer than in midlife sexuality.

TRANSITION: THE KEY TO MASTERING MIDLIFE SEXUALITY

In adolescence, under the influence of cascading sex hormones, expectations are grand and limitations few. The sense of sexual possibilities is best summed up by Buzz Lightyear's gallant cry in *Toy Story:* "To infinity—and beyond!"

Then comes "first" adulthood. Sex is fast and furious. We flex our muscles, find careers, girlfriends, and/or wives. Settling down, we find our rhythm and hit our stride. For years this feels right, but then the rhythm begins to feel like a rut. We begin to expect the expected and view change as a hassle. A nagging fear presents itself: we already are all that we'll ever be. And what we are doesn't feel like nearly enough.

But usually between the ages of 35 and 55, things happen that can change all that. To his horror, a man might find he can't muster an erection, or his wife leaves him, or he gets fired or a parent dies, or any number of other personal and professional bombshells explode in his life. He staggers, falls, gets up, and staggers some more. Wonderfully, however, he gets a chance to reorient himself, to change, and grow. That's the beauty of midlife. And midlife sexuality.

It's within our power to sail into our second adulthood better adjusted, happier, and more fulfilled than ever before. But first we have some work to do. We need to stop blaming others for our own confusion. We need to confront what's going on in our body, our mind, and our emotions. It's not easy, but the rewards are huge.

THRIVING PHYSICALLY AT MIDLIFE

To resist some of what's going on physically in the general neighborhood of forty to fifty is natural. Hair grays or thins. The old energy and strength ain't what they used to be. Body fat surges (especially around the midsection). And if that's not enough, sexual changes creep into the picture. The urge for ejaculation may decrease, along with the distance of each spurt. Erections can change too: Old Faithful may not be as stiff, may not stand as high, may need more time or help to firm up. Those are common changes experienced by many men. But impotence is another matter; feared by many in midlife, it is not at all something to be expected or accepted (more in *Impotence*). If midlife is the time of sexual change, it's also a time for reinvigoration.

Here are eight steps to insure your sexy body retains its glow:

Eat Well

Along with exercise, good nutrition is the best all-around plan for keeping fit, sexually and otherwise. Yet despite all the documented benefits of eating well, men are still nutrition cowboys. Compared with women, we eat less fruits and vegetables and more fat, are less likely to keep a lid on sugar consumption, and tend to drink more coffee.[107] But eating well is just too easy, too smart, and too enjoyable to ignore. Same goes for vitamins, minerals, and herbs. Consult the *Nutrition* chapter for specifics on how to lay the foundation for good sex now and in years to come.

Exercise

It's the universally-agreed-upon anti-aging miracle. As discussed in the *Exercise* chapter, exercise comes in many forms, but can be divided into three basic areas: aerobic, strength-training, and stretching. Ideally, you're doing some of each to maximize stamina and endurance and keep your body and mind fresh, clear, and disease-free. Being a chip-munching couch potato will not only eventually catch up to you with weight gain, it could very well affect your sexual performance too. So get moving. Get limber. And stay strong and healthy and satisfied.

Stop Smoking

If the health of your lungs and heart isn't reason enough to stop smoking, consider your sexuality. The possible consequences include reduced fertility, reduced ejaculate, and even impotence: nicotine and its by-products have been linked to reduced sperm count, reduced sperm movement, and altered sperm shape (which may cause birth defects).[108] Because smoking causes penile blood vessel constriction, reducing blood flow to the penis, erections may suffer. So much for the sexy image of smoking.

Go Easy On Drugs and Alcohol

Hey, good drinks, good times, donworryaboudit, right? Well, maybe. But put this in the mix: alcohol has been linked with ED, or erectile dysfunction.[109] The fact is, alcohol is a central nervous system depressant. So how much is okay? Not too many doctors argue about a drink or even two per day, but certainly if you experience a sexual problem you should ask yourself if alcohol might be involved, and try doing without it while you find out. Recreational drugs also carry risks. There are no rules or cautions that apply to everyone, however, so ask a health professional you trust for specific advice for you.

Have Regular Medical Examinations

Men are notorious for a cavalier attitude toward health care ("Annual checkup? Who, me?"). And throughout first adulthood they're more likely to get away with it. But in midlife, the risks multiply. For example, prostate and other cancers are much easier to reverse if caught early. Skipping annual exams becomes more risky at midlife and beyond.

Explore Alternatives to Prescription Medications

Midlife tends to be a high-stress period in a man's life leading to various physical and psychological problems. Medications can help but they carry the risk of side effects, such as antidepressants that reduce sexual desire,[110] or heart disease medication that can substantially raise the risk of impotence.[111] Your doctor or a certified herbalist can suggest alternatives that are more sex-friendly.

Take Responsibility For Self-Care

Do you? If not, see the *Penis, Testicles*, and *Prostate* chapters to find out how and why to pay attention to the health of your genitals.

Consider Hormone Replacement Therapy

Is male menopause for real? More and more researchers say yes. Is it the same as a female menopause? Obviously not: in menopause, women lose their reproductive capacity, while men can sire babies for decades longer. But how about irritability and hot flashes and the famous hormonal shifts and the rest—do they apply to men too? No consensus exists on the subject, but some would answer yes.

The increasingly popular subject of hormones and their effects is covered in detail in *Hormones*. But we'll take a quick look here because hormones play a major role in the physical and emotional changes during a man's middle years.

Produced in the endocrine system, hormones are chemical messengers that circulate through the bloodstream, influencing growth, sexual energy, digestion, and more. The level of some hormones decrease throughout life, and in some men they dwindle to levels where their sexual performance suffers. In the past ten to twenty years, doctors have begun testosterone (male hormone) replacement, a corresponding therapy to the more widespread practice of estrogen (female hormone) replacement in women. While some men have responded well, with reports of increased sexual desire and performance, researchers caution that higher levels of testosterone have been associated with prostate cancer. Further research is being done now, and results will impact the future of the practice.

THRIVING MENTALLY AT MIDLIFE

You're nobody's fool. You know the score: time—1; your ability to stop it—0. Okay. Running home to Mommy won't cut it. So when the going gets tough—mentally—the tough get going. The time is now. The subject is your sexual desire and performance at midlife—and your attitudes about them. Here are five good attitudes to consider.

Connect and Communicate

How many new male friends have you made in the last year, two years, five years? If you're like many men, the answer is: not many. As time goes on, we need more, not fewer male friends, especially those who are going through the same things we are. A friend who is able to discuss more than sexual conquests is invaluable; so is a men's group. Some women consider men to be communication-impaired. Prove them wrong. Be a pioneer. When it comes to talking about sex with your lover or someone else you trust, be honest. Try it. You'll like it.

Stop Blaming

Whoa, now here's a big one. Some psychologists say we project outward all the unconscious feelings we're unable to consciously face in ourselves. Like anger. Try to stop projecting it. Try feeling anger in your body. (Where is it happening? In your chest? In your gut?). It's tough, and you may need the help of a therapist to do it. But it's a giant step in midlife, and very liberating. Think of it as an express train to intimacy and its garden of sensual delights.

Re-educate Yourself

The times they are a-changing—again. In some ways, men are where women were twenty years ago in terms of exploring their changing role in a changing world. Men need to keep an open mind and learn new ways of being, working, fathering...and making love.

Have Courage

All of this sounds easy on paper, but it's not easy in life. Some of it is total exploration. No guarantees. Sometimes no lifeline. But courage is traditionally a strong suit for males. Warriors need it and so do men trying to figure out which way is up in midlife. The good news is there are plenty of success stories around. In this book and others. In the cafe down the street and the office down the hall.

Have Faith...

...in yourself and your abilities. Anyone, for instance, who has experienced impotence knows how tough it is to live with. And they know firsthand the wisdom of FDR's advice, "The only thing we have to fear is fear itself." When you're ready for sex that's based in intimacy instead of performance, you'll find a way to satisfaction. You can count on that.

THRIVING EMOTIONALLY AT MIDLIFE

In an essay by Carl Jung, he referred to statistics that reveal men tend to get depressed approaching the age of forty.[112] Other emotions now associated with male midlife include anxiety and irritability—and for those successfully dealing with it all, exhilaration and fulfillment.

Midlife presents a double-whammy for men. Whether you're a super-achieving urban corporate leader or an unassuming rural teacher, the troubling prospect in midlife is the same: limitations. We sense that life is no longer unlimited, along with the realization that we're not as strong as we once were. It's not hard to see why depression becomes more common for men in this time of their lives. And the typical social upheavals in work and family life produce increased levels of stress as well. Needless to say, it can be a challenge to a man's sex life.

Emotions are important keys to remaining stable and making successful midcourse corrections. Men are notorious for being less interested in the emotional side of life, and certainly less interested in communicating about them. But in midlife, they hold important answers to the questions we sometimes desperately ask. Here, then, are four great ways to let feelings help rather than hinder your critical voyage through middle life.

Accept your Emotions

This is the critical first step in integrating emotions into winning midlife sexuality. But it's a lot easier to say than do. Many men ignore or deny emotions of all kinds that complicate their perceived role as tough, focused breadwinner and sex machine. Focusing on emotions can be threatening, embarrassing, or annoying, or all three at once.

Feelings are the key to intimacy, and intimacy is the key to great sex, in midlife and anytime. In fact, one important finding in Shere Hite's report on male sexuality was how many men stressed the importance of emotions in a sexual relationships at this time of their lives.[113]

Of course, not all emotions are pleasurable. But the stronger the impulse to ignore them, the more important to address them. It's shocking to discover that your lover, or a close friend, or trained therapist can actually know more about what you're feeling than you do. Being open to exactly that helps you find out what you really want and need, sexually and otherwise.

Neutralize Stress

Not many things kill good sexual intentions instantly as surely as does stress. Stress-diluted desire can all too easily transform a fine, quivering erection into a shriveled shadow of itself. Stress in itself, stress in reaction to stress, stress-based ailments—the whole business is bad news for sex and health. The good news is that there's no reason to consider stress as bad luck. There are reasons for it, sometimes many reasons, and also many techniques for effectively leaving stress behind.

Taking action against it is especially important in midlife. First, as mentioned above, stressful events tend to cluster at this time of life. Secondly, extended bouts of stress can have a cumulative effect on your body, producing lowered immunity, high blood pressure, or headaches,[114] none of which bode well for sex.

Exercise is a terrific antidote, and there are many suggestions in that chapter.

Cultivate Presence in Place of Fear

Because the chips can seem stacked against you at this time, fear can easily slink into your life. Then, maybe after one drink too many, or a long stretch of overtime, or being with a new lover for the first time in years, your mind is willing but your penis isn't. Then fear becomes a self-fulfilling prophecy, with one sexual failure leading to another.

Fear might be nothing more than a message, telling you that it's time to reevaluate your definition of sex. The uncertainty of midlife demands you to take the reins, and move forward purposefully. Fear isn't a bad thing, unless it becomes a self-perpetuating cycle, because it can motivate you to change. You'll find help in transforming fear to presence in practices like meditation, prayer, yoga, and tantric sex.

Defuse anger

In the long run, anger is bad for sex, bad for relationships, and bad for health. Blowing your top occasionally is an understandable safety valve, but if you feel like you've got a short fuse and are angry often, that's a different story. For your own well-being and for those around you, you need to understand what is making you angry, and make constructive changes. Younger men can deal more effectively with the physiological aspect of anger. At midlife, its cumulative effects can cause serious problems. Your heart and blood vessels, for instance, become more vulnerable to the stress of anger. When it has become a habit, anger might feel good, powerful perhaps, but be aware that it might very well be eroding your health and sexual power. In the moment, go for a run, lift some weights, use a punching bag. For the long term, do whatever's necessary, including therapy, to explore your anger and defuse it.

MONOGAMY

The disillusioned divorcé says that monogamy is for the birds.

And he's right: our feathered friends top the list of the world's most monogamous creatures. Up to 90% of bird species are monogamous, compared with around 12% for primates, and 3% for mammals in general.[115] Maybe that's why our pop songs and poetry compare the experience of love to soaring. After all, a monogamous relationship does offer exhilarating heights of intimate and joyful sharing, with sex adding its unique spice and energy to the mix.

The reality, however, is often closer to ground level. We pay a high price for our monogamous ideal: jealousy, envy, guilt, fevered affairs in cheap motels, and maybe most painful of all, the slow demise of love's passion. All of which, however, shouldn't be accepted as inevitable in a couple's journey through life.

THEN AND NOW

How sweet it was! Sizzling sex every day, week in and week out. Ah, those early days of monogamous passion! But then the months blurred, years passed, and so did sexual passion, until it stands at dead low tide, or worse yet, seemingly dried up altogether.

As you probably suspect, sexual steam has cooled in millions of marriages, as formerly passioned lovers put one foot in front of the other, sex falling in the cracks between today's fatigue and tomorrow's mortgage payment. Barry McCarthy, psychologist at American University in Washington D.C., says that 20% of American marriages are having sex less than 10 times a year,[116] a frequency he uses to classify a relationship as "nonsexual." And many more marriages are plodding downhill in sexual ruts, the excitement slowly draining from the same old arousal, foreplay, intercourse, and afterplay.

Sounds bleak, and it certainly can be so. But not necessarily! In fact, the decline of a couple's sexual fire might be right on schedule, preparing them for the next stage of their relationship: *renewal*. After all, the early, energetic thrills are often based in novelty, infatuation, and unreal expectations. As the relationship deepens, and as individuals grow, sex can pave new avenues of personal and interpersonal growth. Too many partners don't recognize this, and get lost in frustrated attempts to manufacture the original fervor, with their partners or otherwise.

That's a typical and mistaken motivation for giving up on monogamous sex. After all, monogamy offers important keys to great sex: the satisfaction of love, security of commitment, regular mutual support, and a healthy release of tensions. Add a desire for growth and don't be surprised if passion reappears in a new guise

> **Six Steps For Nourishing Relationships**
>
> The Short List:
> - Communicate Early and Often
> - Keep a Perspective
> - Stop the Blame Game
> - Get Real
> - Respect Your Partner
> - Seek Help (When You Need It)

altogether, and transports you to pleasures deeper than you knew existed. The key is to approach the process as a couple, uniting personal responsibility with the vast advantages of monogamy.

COMMUNICATE EARLY AND OFTEN

It's true: the prime sexual rejuvenator isn't genital gymnastics. Talking and touching are the power tools here. As daily pressures and responsibilities mount, partners naturally spend less time with each other, and less time talking together (in many cases, just minutes a day). Hey, we're all too busy just remembering to breathe! But left unchecked, that loss of together-time will lead to major gaps in a relationship. Compensating by spending more time with friends, alcohol, masturbation, or separate vacations only further erodes a couple's shared life.

The more you need to talk, the harder it can be to start. Simple solution: take the plunge. Open up. Don't worry if the words don't come out perfectly. It's the effort that counts. More about this in the *Communication* chapter. Suffice it to say that the surest route to renewed intimacy is clearly expressing who you are, and what you want to give and receive, and listening with equal interest to your partner. We're not talking about one-sided demands here, but the magic of connection and open-hearted intimacy.

KEEP A PERSPECTIVE

Remember, waning passion isn't wholly negative, and it certainly isn't irreversible. It could be a priority message: it's time for change. Not of partners, but of positions. Routines. Attitudes. Boredom is a problem only if you refuse to confront it.

No problem, right? After all, everyone is ready for change—especially after monumental marital arguments. Think of it not as the end of the world, just the dawning of a new day. Seize it!

STOP THE BLAME GAME

When your sex isn't sizzling, blame is a one-way ticket to nowhere, as you probably already know. It doesn't even feel good. So why do it? Lose the illusion that blame helps anything. Take responsibility for yourself. What are *you* feeling? What are *you* contributing to the relationship's lack of movement? What specific steps could *you* take on the road to two-sided arousal? These are the starting points that contribute genuine movement in a stalling or stalled marriage.

GET REAL

Accepting the need for change is the first step. Have you experienced some bitter disappointment or emotional pain? That's the need for change calling. Resisting it is what we're all so good at. Even when our comfort level dips, we scuttle around to keep it propped up with old habits—which were the cause of the pain in the first place. Hey, it's time to look at who we are and why, and what we truly want!

Start with your expectations. If you're looking for nothing but a safe emotional harbor, that might be part of your problem. What about life? Its surprises? Its pitfalls? Its challenges and opportunities for growth?

David Schnarch, author of the powerfully insightful book *Passionate Couples*, says that the true health of an emotionally committed relationship involves each partner responding to a fundamental inner need: being yourself. Profound sexual intimacy arises from knowing who you are and expressing it through sex.[117]

RESPECT YOUR PARTNER

Here's some time-tested, common-sense wisdom from relationships that last: never stop respecting your partner, even if it seems like she's the cause of all your troubles. Because she isn't. There are good reasons you became involved with her in the first place. Don't forget them. Work with them. You can rekindle the old spark—and add potent new ones too, but not by trying to tear down her self-esteem.

SEEK HELP

Sooner or later in the course of your relationship, there will likely come a time when you will feel like walking out the door, never to return. Many do so. Should you?

Not lightly. Not out of boredom. Not without looking hard at your motivation. And probably not without good objective advice. After all, you may not be conscious of all your reasons, including the most pressing. A psychologist is trained to see motives in your behavior that you can't, and to help you see them too. Marriage counselors, sex therapists, psychologists— all valuable resources when you need help. Remember, they're not there just to tell you what to do, but rather to help you find your own best course of action. Maybe you should leave your partner, but hopefully you'll be making the right choices for the right reasons. Not just taking the easiest route for running away from yourself. When you begin to recognize the same problems recurring in your life, then you know that you have something to confront in yourself. Be a man. Take hold of your courage and strength and take a look inside. With help if necessary.

GO FOR PLEASURE, NOT PERFORMANCE

You don't start a campfire by lighting a log, right? A fire is built in stages: first twigs, then branches, and when that's ablaze, you throw on the heavy stuff. Same principle here. Start by concentrating on pleasure, not by demanding mind-blowing ecstasy. In fact, try foregoing intercourse altogether. Concentrate on relearning how to touch, how to be in the moment together. Take your time. This is good. When you're ready, move on, but not at

Seven Tips For Revitalizing Sex, The Short List:

- Go for Pleasure, Not Performance
- Try Both Tracks
- Meet Again
- Go for Variety
- Open Your Eyes
- Use the Magic of Massage
- Escape Together!

the expense of what you've learned about enjoying each other's presence, nakedness, and trust. Fear? Not a problem with that foundation.

TRY BOTH TRACKS

Two very different paths beckon: presence and fantasy. What turns you on now? What turns her on? Simple touch, background music, candles? Or hot and heavy, no-holes-barred pornography? Hey, no judgments, just trial and error, tasting this, squeezing that. Ask and reveal. Size up the possibilities. See what works, and what doesn't. Someone's got to do the experimenting, and you're elected. Could be worse!

MEET AGAIN

Remember when it was new? The anticipation? The preparation? The totally focused attention? Some couples like to revisit all that with actual dates. Obviously, strong and unresolved emotional conflicts work against this option. But if you're both interested, go for it—and don't leave your imagination at home. Meet in a roadside bar, a dancing club, or a dimly-lit restaurant. Make exploratory comments and gestures. Kiss her (especially if you're a movie buff) as if for the first time. Like a method actor, find the emotions inside and relate with them. Then let the acting fall away and be in the moment together, rediscovering that incredible spark at the base of your relationship.

GO FOR VARIETY

Try a vibrator. Make love in a chair. Forget the underwear. With a base of good communication, experimentation can be a big part of revitalizing monogamy. And it's fun too! Masturbate together in the living room. Oil up and slide around belly to back. Try some phone sex. You get the idea.

OPEN YOUR EYES

While kissing. While having an orgasm. David Schnarch presents a strong alternative to the widely accepted technique of "sensate focus," concentrating on sensations to nourish a couple's sexuality: the more partners become differentiated (more truly themselves) the happier their relationship will be, and the more profound their sexuality will become.[118] He calls for open eyes to encourage emotional involvement, which resonates with the main theme of the book mentioned earlier, *Passionate Couples*. Sex as maximized sensation works against emotional connection. And if there's one thing the early days of a relationship point out, it's that sex plus emotions equals true passion in bed.

USE THE MAGIC OF MASSAGE

Explore the fine line between massage and erotic massage. Or use both. Massage is a perfect transition between the rough-and-tumble of daily life and the luxuriant timelessness of making love. Literally rub the tensions away. Breathe deeply. Sense with your fingers. Light a candle. Play soft music. Use exotic essential oils. Feel yourself come back to the present. If the moment is right, for both of you, move on to more erogenous intent, and let the massage be foreplay. Move into sex. Or not. Don't be afraid to talk, to share feelings. This is high-level togetherness; allow the intimacy to take you where it will.

ESCAPE TO THE ISLANDS

We're talking second honeymoon here. Rediscovering each other. Tell your boss you'll see him later. Park the kids with Aunt Mary. Get yourselves to the plane or ship and go!

Consider the possibilities. Hiking through the edelweiss in the Swiss Alps. Eating pineapples on the beach in Maui. What's your pleasure? An all-inclusive setup where everything is provided for you? Or renting a flat for a week in London where you can go out and find a different restaurant every night? Go wherever your two hearts lead you. If it's been too long since you've been alone, invest in your future and get back together in style!

MONOGAMY IN THE WORLD

Daniel and Beth work hard. It took them fifteen years to pay off their college loans. Then they started salting away money for their kids' education, which they felt good about. What felt less good, however, was that they were starting to snap at each other over seemingly trivial matters like who cleans up after dinner or weeds the flower beds. And they were finding less time for sex.

They knew something had to change, but didn't know what. Daniel decided they needed a breath of fresh air. He stopped by a travel agency and booked them on a Caribbean cruise. When he announced this second honeymoon to Beth, she initially objected to the expense, but soon began looking forward to the departure date.

Two months later, they were snorkeling in St. John, the cruise's first stop. Beth couldn't stop thinking about the previous night. It was their first night at sea. They had started the evening with a red snapper dinner. Then they had a glass of wine under starlight on the top deck, and danced under a disco light till midnight. When they got back to their stateroom, Daniel kissed her with a passion she hadn't felt in years. She responded in kind. He suggested the she lie on the edge of the bed, something he had never done, and proceeded to excite her with oral sex techniques she had also never experienced. She felt like she was floating, which of course she was.

The rest of the cruise was similarly satisfying. When they returned home, both felt a new lease on life. It inspired them to be more open about their feelings and frustrations. They often look at their photo album of the cruise, and are planning another one next year. Their second honeymoon wasn't the answer to all their problems, but it certainly was a giant step in the right direction.

NUTRITION

Want a lifetime of great sex?

Learn how to eat right.

Good eating and exercise are the ticket to peak sexual fitness. Medical or recreational drugs can stimulate a man, but over the long haul they're a prescription for dependence and side effects.

You want energy and stamina. All-systems-go. Eating right may not be the most dramatic approach, but it's one of the surest and most reliable. Hopefully you've discovered that already. Too often it takes a heart attack to awaken the nutritionally-handicapped male. And while for one man the wake-up call is a life-threatening health problem, for another it's a lifestyle-threatening sexual problem. For health and longevity—and sexual fitness— why wait until the horse has left the barn?

Habits die hard. Too often we obey weird macho signals that make us stall and deny and weaken and clog. Visit a doctor? No time! Talk to him about a sexual problem? Hah! We're too busy putting one foot in front of the other in a high-stress world, awash in the stream of advertising when not guided by inherited and unhealthy tastes. Fortunately, good solid nutrition can help—with your health, your peace of mind, and your sex life. Read on to discover how food, nutritional supplements, and herbs can lead to creating and maintaining great sexual performance and satisfaction.

BUILD THE GROUNDWORK FOR GREAT SEX

Here's the key: vigorous and lasting sexual fitness arise from optimal overall health. From brain chemistry to erections, sexual response is a complex interaction of nerves, hormones, organs, and other bodily miracles. From one point of view, it's *all* chemistry, which may not be the most romantic slant on sexual desire, performance, and potency, but it's an essential one. The foundation of a healthy body is created and nourished with the components of food, which simply echoes the old ditty from 1969: *you are what you eat.*

If you're tempted to shrug your shoulders and joke about feeling like another greasy burger, think about the fact that *millions* of your peers suffer from high blood pressure, high cholesterol, low sexual desire, or impotence.

And don't expect the miracles of modern medicine to save you in the long run from years of disrespecting your body's needs. Get on the fast track to health and sexual fitness. Eat right—now.

FOUR REASONS TO UPGRADE YOUR NUTRITION

Desire

Today, low sexual desire is a common complaint—in men and women. One often-overlooked cause is what passes for three daily meals today. In his book *Sexual Nutrition*, Dr. Morton Walker spotlights the distinction between high-level and low-level wellness. What some people call health may be the absence of disease, but it really treads the line between sickness and health, and might more accurately be called *low-level health*.[119]

Living without the spark of sexual excitation or fulfillment could itself be a symptom of life in that gray area. Dr. Walker attributes an imbalanced diet and refined foods as important causes.

If you're feeling low energy in general or in your sex life in particular, look at what you eat. A poor diet is easier to change than other causes of low-level health like environmental pollution, and improving what you eat can help you thrive despite stressors beyond your direct ability to change.

Performance

Sexual performance is a hot button for most men, to say the least. Performance not in the sense of acting, of course, but the physiological process of erection and ejaculation. Combined with the physical aspect are emotions and attitudes, all pointing to the same reality: you want to be able to satisfy and be satisfied. Being unable to perform is a tough pill to swallow.

To a large degree, it's all about free-flowing *energy*. The initial interest, the stir in your shorts, the embrace, the emotional afterglow—everything. This is particularly stressed in Eastern traditions, where health and sex are tied directly to your overall energy, your *chi*, and its flow through your body. Biochemically your energy comes from food. Sure, various stimulants can rev you up, but the royal road to long-term reliable health and sexual energy is a good diet.

Another basic determinant of male sexual performance is circulation, or blood flow. Your penis swells into an erection because its spongy tissues fill with blood (as detailed in the *Penis* chapter), which makes it a story about sex and the heart, but not the kind with a fella sitting on a barstool cryin' into his beer. Blood flow is the vital connection between the astonishing organic pump in your chest, the condition of your blood vessels, and stiff erections. There are foods, nutritional supplements, and herbs which can promote that teamwork, and you'll find them below.

Healing and Prevention

Major studies reveal the astonishing power of food to promote health and prevent the most serious illnesses and conditions of our time, including infertility, impotence, erectile dysfunction, and prostate cancer.

For example, *The New England Journal of Medicine* reported that adding *one serving* of fruits or vegetables a day reduced the risk of stroke by 40%, more than cholesterol-lowering drugs.[120] What does that have to do with you? Plenty, if you like erections. Arteriosclerosis, or thickening and hardening of the arteries, is caused by deposits of fatty plaque (which includes cholesterol) in the arteries. It reduces blood flow and can cause strokes and heart attacks. The blood vessels supplying the penis are not exempt. In fact, one recent study found a link between high cholesterol levels and erectile dysfunction.[121] Bottom line: eat right and rise to the occasion.

Fertility

In general, men today produce less sperm than their ancestors. All factors contributing to the difference are unknown. Likely causes include environmental pollutants, stress, and faulty diets. Deficiency of zinc in the body can lead to reduced sperm counts, as well as impotence and inflammation of the prostate gland[122]—crucial information when we consider that zinc is deficient in the soils of thirty-two states in America.[123] We'll look more closely at this important question for fathers-to-be. Right now let's see how the preceding overview relates to your kitchen table and bedroom.

FOOD FOR SEX

Find the combination of foods producing good energy and good circulation, and you're supporting great sex. Our focus here is not spiking desire or performance with save-me-if-you-can stimulants. Rather, we're looking for the foods and other nutrients that provide vital everyday wellness—so you're fit for everyday sexual magic. We'll start with the basics—food groups, nutrient analysis, high octane sex fuel, and so forth.

Sex is a workout. Breathing quickens, blood pressure rises, muscles contract and release, etc. These reactions, along with those in male genitals, require a complex set of inner reactions. How well you respond is conditioned by your intake from basic food groups. Basic food groups? That's right, we're starting at the beginning here. A quick run-through of nutrition fundamentals will allow a better understanding of the latest tips on sexual nutrition.

A simple pie chart once summed up general knowledge of the four basic food groups, with slices of meat, dairy, fruits/vegetables, and cereals/grains.

Then in 1992, the government released new guidelines in the form of a Food Guide Pyramid, four tiers illustrating the ideal daily consumption from each food group. The bottom, and largest, section contains bread, cereal, rice and pasta. Following is the next-higher level of vegetables and fruits; then meat, poultry, fish, beans, eggs, and nuts and beans, milk, yogurt, and cheese; and finally the top and smallest section, fats, oils, and sweets. Okay, sounds reasonable.

The point was to maximize American health. But critics have pointed out that the American male's pot belly is growing nonetheless, and new research shows that midsection fat is associated with a higher risk of diabetes, cancer, and heart disease.[124] Our immediate question is, how does that affect America's erection?

GETTING TO THE HEART OF THE MATTER

Despite charts and pyramids and diets of all descriptions, one in three Americans today is seriously overweight.[125] And almost one in four has high blood pressure.[126] Those statistics land us in cardiovascular territory— blood circulation, which, as we've seen, has a direct impact on male sexuality. To understand the functioning of heart and blood vessels and penis, we need to look at macronutrients, or the building blocks of food: protein, carbohydrate, and fat.

More and more forward-thinking doctors and health experts are looking critically at the official food pyramid. They see health benefits of certain kinds of carbohydrates, protein, and fat, and the proportions in which they're eaten. The right combination of these make for a strong cardiovascular system, with less clogging cholesterol, optimum weight, and balanced, readily-available energy. This sounds like perfect contributions to sexual fitness too.

New nutritional trends are emerging; we'll explore them now.

EIGHT FIT-FOR-SEX EATING TIPS

The good news is that you don't have to choose between a platter of steak or a bowl of bird food. Fit-for-Sex eating includes a broad range of eating pleasures. It's a create-your-own-success story for health and sex. For simplicity, here are eight steps for new pleasures in the dining room and the bedroom.

Rethink Carbohydrates

Critics question the strong emphasis on the high carbohydrate base of the standard food pyramid. Barry Sears, in his book *The Zone*, maintains that the body converts excess carbohydrates to fat. He also counsels for a new balance of complex carbohydrates, protein, and fat in every meal and snack. Critics maintain that the higher-protein aspect can lead to an acidic condition in the body or even kidney damage.[127]

There is a growing consensus that complex carbohydrates (listed below) should be emphasized, and simple carbohydrates like refined sugar and flour should be minimized. While this isn't exactly late-breaking news, if you're like most guys, there's still a lot of that refined stuff headed to your plate and waistline.

Add to your plate: whole grains, legumes, vegetables, fruits.

Cut down or eliminate: refined rice, refined grain pasta, bread, bagels, cereals, etc.

Choose Healthy Fats

Big benefits are yours in re-examining dietary fat. Are you excited? You should be, because you can choose between foods that promote wellness and those that promote sickness by damaging your cells (in the service of increased product shelf life) and wreak havoc in your sex life.

While the standard food pyramid calls for minimal fat consumption, it doesn't differentiate between *types* of fat. Eating too little fat is counterproductive; all kinds play a positive role. But one group, the *essential fatty acids* (EFA's) are especially important for two reasons: 1) they do a lot of good in your cardiovascular system (and joints and skin), and 2) your body can't make its own. The recommended oils and food below insure that you're covered (including the much-publicized Omega 3's and 6's).

On the negative side, *hydrogenated fats* (or trans-fatty acids) are increasingly called villains. These oils are produced with added hydrogen, which solidifies them and increases product shelf life. But wait a minute, what sounds more important to you: shelf life or sex life? Dr. Andrew Weil, in *Eight Weeks to Optimum Health*, recommends avoiding the many food products containing hydrogenated fats.[128] Check your own cabinets—you'll be surprised to see how many packages qualify for the heave-ho.

Enjoy: cold-water fish (salmon, mackerel, sardines, herring, tuna), nuts and seeds, most whole grains, soybeans, lean meats, leafy greens, flaxseed oil, wild game, legumes, olive oil, canola oil, evening primrose oil, and black currant oils.

Avoid or minimize: cottonseed oil, margarine, hydrogenated or partially hydrogenated oils (especially prevalent in oil and grain products like salad and cooking oils, breads, crackers, cookies, and pastas). And go easy on fatty animal and dairy products too.

Eat Lean Proteins

Protein is necessary for building new cells, tissues, and hormones, and it also creates energy and regulates fluids. So how much, and what kind, should you eat?

As you've probably guessed, the answer is moderation. Eat too little protein and your energy level can plunge. With too much you can be headed to heart disease or osteoporosis. Also, much has been written about the overuse of growth hormones and antibiotics in the beef and poultry industries. The safest way to avoid any resulting problems is organic meat and poultry.

Maximize: lean beef, poultry, fish, eggs, soybean products (like tofu and tempeh).

Minimize: high-fat beef, high-fat cheese

Say Hello to Fruits and Vegetables

"You're not leaving the table 'til you finish your peas!"

Too many of us still associate vegetables with sitting alone in the kitchen, defiantly staring at a few peas on an otherwise empty plate. Today there are many compelling reasons to change our attitudes toward fruits and vegetables. Collectively they're called phytonutrients: the nutrients in plants. To your defense, there may not have been too many left in those pale green canned peas.

We'll all be hearing a lot about phytonutrients in the future. And with good reason. While they've always been there, researchers are now finding their many important health benefits, and how their lack can be reflected in high-profile diseases like heart disease and cancer. Many are further grouped under another word already much talked about: antioxidants.

Antioxidants neutralize renegade oxygen cells called free radicals, which attract and damage healthy cells. Those previously healthy cells then become free radicals too, and an unhealthy chain reaction builds into disease and/or premature aging. Cholesterol, for instance, goes from good to bad after being altered by free radicals (more about cholesterol below). And just that one example can adversely affect your sexual get-up-and-go.

So eat at least 5-8 servings of fruits and vegetables every day. Broccoli, apples, onions, grapes, tomatoes, carrots, and many others...fresh, in soups, salads, sauces...take your choice. And enjoy the tastes and benefits.

Revise Your Thinking about Cholesterol

Ah, health news. Just when safe guidelines bring peace of mind, new findings advance from the horizon like towering afternoon clouds borne on a swift summer wind.

In short, in the interest of good health and good sex, it's time to revise your thinking about cholesterol, now that it has been linked to erection and prostate problems.

Until recently, the accepted view was simple: eat too many high-fat foods and arteries clog up with cholesterol until blood can't flow properly and chest pains signal a heart attack. In fact, this view is so simple, it's oversimplified.

First, it became clear that there was more than one kind of cholesterol; one was good (HDL), and another was bad (LDL). Good cholesterol helps with important bodily functions, such as producing hormones and repairing injuries to arteries. LDL cholesterol was found to be bad news, especially as related to blood fats called triglycerides in the plaque formations that harden and constrict blood vessels.

Now our view is becoming more refined yet. The *New England Journal of Medicine* notes that most heart attack patients have normal cholesterol levels.[129] In fact, recent studies show elevated levels of homocysteine (an amino acid) as a higher factor for heart attack than cholesterol. Those elevated levels may account for many cases of vascular disease in this country. Since cardiovascular health and male sexuality are related, this should ring some bells. And call for action.

Yes, high levels of cholesterol are cause for concern. And keeping saturated fats and refined carbohydrates to a minimum helps. But here's yet another reason to add more fruits and vegetables to your diet. Folate (or its synthetic version, folic acid) regulates homocysteine levels, which rise after you've eaten animal protein. The richest sources are dark-green leafy vegetables, carrots, cabbage, orange juice, asparagus, beans, wheat germ and okra. Since it takes a lot of those to get enough every day, a supplement can help.

Eat Whole Foods

Eating right means balancing different kinds of foods to get the nutrients you need, but also important is the *quality* of foods. There's plenty of debate about this. One medical reference book says organically produced food has no nutritional advantage over conventionally produced food.[130] Obviously, natural food enthusiasts disagree. They cite nutritional advantages of organic food, and they warn about the long-term toxicity of ingested pesticides, as well as unknown dangers arising from different pesticides combining in our systems.[131] Kathy Keville, author of *Herbs for Health and Healing*, raises the possibility of reduced sperm counts caused by feminine hormone-like material (which lowers male testosterone levels) in pesticides and meat and dairy products too.[132]

Take Vitamin and Mineral Supplements

Once upon a time, good food supplied all necessary vitamins and minerals. No more. Depleted soils, polluted air, and high-speed/high-stress lives make it difficult to get all the nutrients we need. When possible, eat organic food. And for optimum health and sexual fitness, consider daily vitamin and mineral supplements. Below is a list of micronutrients (another name for vitamins and minerals) related to sexual health.

Zinc: Casanova reputedly ate many oysters every day. They contain twenty times more zinc than any other food.[133] Case closed.

On a more scientific note, most of the body's zinc is stored in the testes, where it plays a major role in powering arousal, erections, sperm count, and prostate health. But maintaining an adequate supply in the body is difficult due to refined foods, depleted zinc in soils, consumption of alcohol, and aging (less is absorbed from foods). Good dietary sources of zinc, beyond oysters, include meat, fish, nuts, seeds, spinach, parsley, collards, peas, whole wheat, rye, and oats.

Vitamin E: Considered by some to be the most important vitamin for sex, vitamin E promotes healthy blood flow, hormone production, and sex gland maintenance. Therefore, this makes it important for sexual desire and response, as well as for prostate health. Good dietary sources include wheat germ oil, sunflower seeds, safflower oil, eggs, peanuts, and almonds.

Selenium: This mineral helps with vitamin E absorption, and is a potent antioxidant in itself. It also acts as a natural chelating agent, which binds with unhealthy materials in the body (such as heavy metals) and moves them out. Selenium deficiency has been linked to prostate cancer. Foods rich in selenium are herring, wheat germ, brazil nuts, butter, whole wheat bread, oats, shrimp, oysters, and red Swiss chard.

Vitamin C: An important antioxidant, vitamin C promotes well-being and prevents bodily damage on a cellular level. More vitamin C is required as the body ages, and an adequate supply is needed for continuing sexual energy. Foods high in this vitamin are rosehips, red and green peppers, kale, parsley, citrus fruit, strawberries, and broccoli.

Vitamin A: This vitamin is one of your testicles' best friends. Besides keeping testicles healthy, it is a necessary component of sex hormones, and helps maintain high sperm count. Good sources are liver, carrots, dried apricots, kale, spinach, fish liver oil, and eggs.

Phosphorus: Widespread in the body, phosphorus has been linked to the production of sex hormones and the maintenance of sexual desire. Foods rich in phosphorus have reputed aphrodisiac qualities in Chinese and

European lore, appearing in the form of curries, hot sauces, and truffles. Other food sources include wheat germ and pumpkin seeds.

B Vitamins: The B vitamin complex helps produce testosterone, and has been used to treat male infertility. The component vitamins are also necessary for optimum nerve function and energy level, two building blocks of vital sexual functioning. One of the B vitamins, PABA, has been used to correct Peyronie's disease, which can cause a curved penis and subsequently painful erections. The richest sources of the B vitamins complex is found in brewers yeast, liver, wheat germ, wild rice, and eggs.

Discover the Power of Herbs

There's a fine line between medicinal herbs and food; in fact there's often no line at all.

Before the 1930's, when broad-spectrum antibiotics first appeared in the modern world, medicine in America was largely an herbal affair. But then powerful modern drugs quickly supplanted the tradition of natural herbal remedies.

Today, however, many Americans are reconsidering pharmaceutical drugs and their potentially hazardous side effects and high cost. Herbal remedies are gaining in popularity due to their relative safety, affordability, and different approach to healing.

Pharmaceutical drugs target symptoms. And while they often eliminate them efficiently, they can interfere with the functions and balance of bodily systems, causing adverse reactions ranging from discomfort to death. Some would argue that drugs sacrifice the safety of whole plants for the power, and the profit, of patentable synthetic versions.

A heated debate between natural and pharmaceutical medicine has arisen. Today an increasingly popular middle ground combines the best of both methods. Following is an overview of herbs that stabilize, energize, supercharge, and otherwise help male sexuality. Consult your doctor or an herbalist to find which might work for you in addition to, or instead of, medical drugs.

HERBS FOR SEXUAL FITNESS

In China, Ginseng has a long history of stimulating male sexual desire, mostly in men over 40. It is said to restore desire by raising testosterone levels and overall energy. Don't look for instant results, however.

Proponents claim that only after taking ginseng over a period of months will the benefit be realized, but it's worth the wait because sexual desire *and* stamina are improved. Scientific studies confirm the results with animals; critics note the absence of clinical tests with humans. The best way to know for yourself? Try some. The American species is hard to find, since most of it gets exported to Asia. Try a tonic with the root in the bottle, found in your closest urban Chinatown, or the extract sold in your local health food store.

Physicians in the Ayurvedic tradition are equally enthusiastic about an herb called *ashwaganda*, known for enhancing sexual desire and performance.

Gingko has become famous for its ability to stimulate brain function and boost memory. It accomplishes that by strengthening circulation, which, as we've seen, can boost sexual performance. So gingko is increasingly used as a remedy for impotence. Again, it's not an instant fix; results usually appear in one to two months. James Duke, author of *Nature's Pharmacy*, notes one study in which 78% of men experienced improvement with erectile problems caused by an atherosclerotic penile artery.[134] Don't expect an herbal tea to do the trick, since fifty pounds of leaves from the ginkgo tree produce only one pound of the extract recommended to have a sexual effect. Fortunately, that extract is readily available in health food stores.

Yohimbe is an herbal impotence remedy derived from the bark of an African tree. It stimulates erections and prolongs them as well. But more side effects are reported than is usual for herbal remedies. Even some herbalists recommend taking pharmaceutical versions, which isolate a compound called yohimbine. Studies show that it can correct impotence problems stemming from physical or psychological causes, but you'll need a prescription, which is a good idea because there are some medical conditions with which yohimbine shouldn't be combined.

Other herbs and spices have reputations as sexual enhancers: anise, cardamom, cinnamon, ginger, oats, and the essential oils clary sage, rose, and jasmine.

Saw Palmetto is a small palm tree native to Florida. Many men have been introduced to herbal remedies because of this herb and the relief it brings from their prostate gland's enlargement. That growth is due to hormonal changes, specifically those related to testosterone, which in an aging man can turn into a related hormone called dihydrotestosterone (DHT). DHT can cause prostate cells to multiply, and the prostate gland to enlarge. Symptoms then include frequent or difficult urination.

Both saw palmetto and the pharmaceutical drug Proscar can prevent testosterone from becoming DHT. According to a recent study, the herb was more effective, and faster, in relieving prostate enlargement symptoms. Also 5% of the men on Proscar suffered from decreased libido, ejaculatory disorders, or impotence, while no such side effects were reported with saw palmetto. Its cost was approximately one-third that of Proscar.[135] Other studies in America and Europe confirm the herb's power and safety.

Other foods and herbs linked to prostate health are **Pygeum, Pumpkin Seeds, Licorice,** and **Stinging Nettle**. The herb **Echinacea** boosts immunity and helps clear prostate and urinary infections.

ORAL SEX

1998 was a banner year for oral sex. It emerged from America's bedroom and landed in the living room. Week after week national politics focused on intimate details of a presidential tryst, with one central question prevailing: is oral sex really sex? Politics being what it is, the question was never really answered.

The tumult extended as well to the world of scientific research. The editor of a venerable research publication, the *Journal of the American Medical Association*, was promptly fired for publishing a study about what was, and was not, considered to be sex by a group of college men and women. (For the record, the 1991 survey showed that 59% of the students did not consider having oral-genital contact as having "had sex."[136])

Of course the legal ramifications of oral sex extend far beyond our nation's capital. Did you know, for instance, that it's still illegal in nine states for a married couple to engage in oral sex in their own bedroom?[137]

So much for the public arena. But what about you? How do you feel about oral sex? Do your feelings about it relate to your fitness for sex? Obviously that depends on your partner. If she wants it and you don't, or vice versa, that could cause a wrinkle. But if you both find it distasteful, then there's no problem. Not to worry, you won't find any effort here to convince you otherwise.

If you appreciate the art of oral-genital sex, you have plenty of company!

MANY LIKE IT HOT

Technically, a woman using her mouth or tongue on a man's penis is called *fellatio*. A man using his mouth or tongue on a woman's vulva is *cunnilingus*. Those are the official names; they certainly don't convey much about the fine points and pleasure involved with licking, kissing, and sucking, in this intimate area. The subject of oral sex is wide—as wide as an ocean of desire.

The subject is hot. Or cold, depending on whom you ask. Some men and women consider it an unspeakable and intolerable offense to civilization. Others can't get enough and eagerly await the next opportunity to partake.

Widely reported polls show that despite what Americans say or don't say publicly, many like giving and receiving oral sex. Even in the generally conservative findings of a recent University of Chicago sex survey, over two-third of women aged 18-44 said they found *receiving* oral sex very or some-what appealing; 40% of those 45-59 said the same. Over 80% of the men 18-44 liked receiving it; over 60% of the 45-59 group liked it too.[138] Though the percentages were smaller, the clear majority of both younger groups reported *giving* oral sex very or somewhat appealing. In a different study of married couples aged 25 or younger, 90% reported experience with oral sex.[139]

One may conclude, therefore, that many Americans are enjoying it. Are you? If you're interested in trying it, or refining your style, then please read on. All others should skip to the next chapter.

ORAL SEXUAL FITNESS

In a way, oral sex epitomizes some of the challenges of sex overall. It can be intimidating the first time. You may be working against some pretty deeply ingrained attitudes, and some deep emotional issues can pop up regarding the vulnerability of your position (and hers). These are prime areas where you and your lover can evolve together in the melting pot of intimacy. As already mentioned, it doesn't appeal to everyone. Being open to new possi-bilities, willing to learn and communicate, and caring enough to be fully involved with the emotional life of your partner and yourself—these have been undervalued aspects of sexual fitness for too long, and are all in the foreground of oral sex.

That said, why even consider touching mouths to genitals in the first place?

SIX REASONS FOR ORAL SEX

Primo Satisfaction

First of all, you don't need a reason to enjoy oral sex. If both parties are interested, that's reason enough. But there are other reasons you may not have considered, and may want to consider in the future.

One fact we'll return to more than once is that many a woman absolutely loves a man's mouth on her clitoris, and to a lesser but still considerable extent, his tongue in her vagina. Many women consider it the preferred choice in foreplay. In fact, many women find the physical sensations of cunnilingus more intense than intercourse.

So, the number one reason for putting your mouth on your partner's privates is that it might very well drive her passionately wild.

Birth Control

For young couples—or older ones—wanting to avoid pregnancy, oral sex is a stellar combination of 100% effective contraception plus a heaping helping of pleasure. Of course the obvious assumption there is that sex is more than a reproductive act. Some sexually conservative couples believe that's all it is, which is fine for them. Others believe sex to be a matter of pleasure and health as well, which is fine for them too.

> ### Safe Oral Sex
>
> When a man and a woman decide to engage in oral sex, each should be aware of the dangers of sexually transmitted diseases. Although there is no absolute consensus on the subject, many researchers believe there is danger of contracting the HIV virus orally, as well as hepatitis B, herpes, and other STD's. Unless you have both been tested or are otherwise convinced you're safe, use a condom on yourself and a dental dam (try the flavored varieties!) or other effective barrier on her. As with the rest of sex, being safe is smart, and precautions should be integrated with passion.

After Giving Birth

No, not right afterwards, good sir. But again, depending on a couple's preferences, if both partners feel the erotic urge and the desire to share it before her vagina has fully recovered, oral sex can be welcome intimacy. Needless to say, it's her call on this one.

Instant Intimacy

Sometimes passion runs high but time is short. If circumstances work against even an intercourse quickie, there's always oral sex! More likely you'll be receiving here. If you've got a gem of a woman who understands, lucky you!

During Menstruation

Okay, so this option isn't for everyone. But remember, menstruation isn't a steady affair, nor does it necessarily diminish desire. So if she's clean and ready and intercourse isn't in the cards, go oral!

An ED Alternative

The truck driver's booming voice delivers his street wisdom to an elderly man helping him unload. "Can't get it up anymore? No problem, you can always get your tongue up!" Well, in his own way he captures an important truth. When a man, for whatever reason, experiences erectile dysfunction (no erection), sex doesn't have to end. Remember, oral sex is so satisfying to many women they prefer it over intercourse. You can still be intimate in many ways, and oral sex is one of the most powerful.

Age, injury, circulatory problems, etc.? No problem! You can always use your tongue (after consulting with your doctor)!

EIGHT TIPS FOR DRIVE-HER-CRAZY CUNNILINGUS

Proceed Slowly

There she is, legs spread, trusting you with the most private part of her body. How do you begin? *Gently.* In fact don't just slide down after a token hug and kiss. Before stimulating her down below, connect with her up above. Take your time. Gradually work your way down with kisses or a tongue bath for her chest, belly, inner thighs, or wherever else she likes. When you get between her legs, keep the pace slow. Whether you're exploring for the first time or have been here before, she'll appreciate your care. A woman's clitoris, though in some ways comparable to a penis, is more sensitive. After she's warmed up you can apply more pressure, if she so desires. You'll need to discover her preferences by trial and error, or through her words, sounds, and movement. But that's half the fun, and more than half the excitement!

Get Positioned for the Long Haul

One thing to keep in mind as you go down on her: you might be there awhile. Like twenty or thirty minutes or more. So get comfortable. There's no poetry in her writhing in passion while you're in cramped muscle agony. If she's lying in bed and you're between her legs, find the right combination of lying or kneeling and change between them. Maybe you could be on the floor with her on the edge of the bed. And for that matter, neither of you has to be in bed! Maybe she's draped over the grand piano with your mouth between her legs and your fingers playing Beethoven's Moonlight Sonata. Whatever! Just remember to be comfortable.

Use All Relevant Territory

Stay in exploration mode. You've got a compact but varied erotic landscape at close range. First there's the pubic mound, above her genitals per se. Don't be surprised if she rubs this while you're busy below. If not, you can do it for her, before or during your mouth play. Take a good look at her vulva; it consists of outer lips, inner lips, clitoris, urethra opening, and vagina. All relevant. All sensitive. All you need to flood her with ecstasy. Don't be surprised if she wants you to focus on her clitoris, at least when she's in the home stretch.

Use All Oral Options

Your mouth is a versatile instrument, capable of much more than forming words. You've got lips. A tongue. And many ways to combine them to build her passion.

Let's start with your lips. Use them to kiss, nuzzle, suck, wiggle, and so on. When her excitement builds, you can try giving her clitoris a gentle suck, combined with a gentle swipe of the tongue. Now's the time to use all your pent-up creativity. Penetrate her vagina with your tongue, pump and slurp a bit. With time you'll discover what she likes best.

Don't Get Lost Down There

Just because you're between her legs physically doesn't mean you should drift into orbit mentally. Stay in touch! Remember you're making love here. Stay intimate. Stay connected. You don't necessarily have to stop talking or making eye contact. When you're done—and she is too—you'll both be ready for a more full-bodied contact, and in all likelihood, astonishing intercourse. So stay tuned!

Add Options

Okay, you've got a great thing going with your lips and tongue. But why stop there? As good as that can be, you can always add another element or two. How about incorporating a vibrator? Or putting an ice cube into your mouth and giving her clitoris a cool surprise? Or dab some peanut butter and jelly on and languorously lap it up. Hey, you've got a home full of surprises available. Surprise her! Surprise yourself!

Enjoy All Your Senses

If this is your first time, you might be surprised by the smells and fluids and sounds coming your way. If a woman is clean and healthy, the smell of her excitement turns many a man on. So give it a chance. If her smell knocks you off your feet, you might suggest she wash up the next time—or offer to do it yourself while you're both relaxing in a tub. Cleanliness is a must-have basic. And of course that goes for you when you're receiving.

As for the sense of hearing, what a blessing! Not only is her voice helpful in guiding you in your efforts, but the whispered moans! Whimpers! Forceful groans! Major league turn-on! As is the sight of her from this unique perspective.

Swivel into 69

Oral sex doesn't have to be one-after-the-other. When you turn so that each of your mouths has access to the other's genitals simultaneously, you're in the classic 69 position. Although some couples find they prefer to concentrate on giving or receiving alone, you owe it to yourself to try this position at least once. Either of you can be on top, or you could try it side by side. With practice you might want to aim for simultaneous orgasms, although too much focus on that can detract from the experience for some. The position is not for everyone, but for some it's the cat's meow.

ORAL SEX FOR YOU

Most of what we have been talking about is giving her pleasure orally. Of course there's nothing wrong with your getting some too. It's not something you can force, needless to say. But if your lover is open to the idea, don't be surprised if she ends up liking it. You can help that outcome by keeping yourself clean down there. Take a cue from the French and try the bidet approach even if you don't have one. Squat in a bathtub, soap up, and rinse your private parts. Just takes a minute and can make all the difference.

Help by explaining, or showing, what you like. Let her know when you're approaching orgasm so she can opt not to take your sperm in her mouth if she prefers. Also mention though that she's only looking at about five calories if it comes to that. And if she really gets into it, mention that there are techniques of positioning her head and breathing through her nose that make deep-throating possible.[140] If she's just into basic licking and sucking, hey, that'll work too!

ORGASM

A few simple muscle spasms. And a pleasure too intense for words. It's called an orgasm and nowhere in the world of sex is there a greater paradox.

For most men the lure of orgasm is the driving force behind sex. Relationships have risen and fallen based on the quality, or absence, of orgasms. Yet they can sometimes amount to little more than a skimpy dribble of pleasure. Heck, they can even be had while asleep. It's kind of funny really, although few men consider orgasms a laughing matter.

Maybe one reason for the seriousness is that like erections, orgasms involve more than the body. Nothing boosts a good orgasm like shared emotion. And nothing detracts more than the tension of negative feelings.

HERE YOU COME

The biomechanics of sperm delivery are described in *Ejaculation* and *Fertility*. But there's something new here. Somewhere in the process of semen delivery comes a *feeling*—orgasm—and a very good feeling at that. The relationship between orgasm and ejaculation is described differently depending on who you ask.

Traditionally in our culture, orgasm and ejaculation have been informally described as occurring simultaneously—ejaculation being the sperm-spurting portion of orgasm.[141] In this view, orgasm is a two-stage event, consisting of semen being readied for launch, and then its launch out of the penis.

Supercharge Your Orgasm

Try your trusty Kegels to intensify orgasms. (If you don't know what they are, see the chapter on Kegels. By contracting your PC muscles you can learn to stop yourself before the point of no return. If you can get to the point of delaying orgasm this way, you might find more intensity to the release itself.

The first stage is called emission; the second, expulsion. Emission consists mainly of preparatory contractions. The prostate, vas deferens ampulla, seminal vesicles, and the penis urethra all contract, sending sperm into the base of the urethra. Then explusion: the pelvic muscles contract, the urethra relaxes, and semen is forcefully ejected from the penis.

Today, however, an alternate view of orgasm is gaining popularity: emission (the contracting phase) is where orgasm starts, and can take place regardless of whether expulsion does. So the pleasure of orgasm can be experienced without arousal-ending ejaculation (which is normally followed by the refractory phase, or rest period where sexual excitement fades and the body readies itself for another orgasm).

By delaying or foregoing ejaculation, sexual excitement remains high, and multiple orgasms for men are possible. This is different from multiple orgasms *with* ejaculation (and short refractory periods) that many younger men can achieve. More about multiple orgasms later.

First let's check in with her.

THE FEMALE VERSION

A woman also experiences physiological changes prior to and with orgasm: an expanding uterus and inner vagina, the outer part of the vagina swelling with blood, and her clitoris receding under its hood. Then she too experiences muscle contractions, locally in her genitals and throughout her body. But from the point of you as her lover, those physiological aspects of orgasm are less important than the fact that she's capable of different kinds of orgasms.

That this topic is still so wrapped in mystery is interesting in itself. But today there's nothing mysterious about many a woman's reaction to missionary-position-only sex. She's likely be frustrated, expecting more, and

Exploring a Clitoris

Female sexual anatomy includes the mysterious (to many men) clitoris, the sensitive little bud atop a woman's vulva. At one point in our fetal development, male and female genitals are exactly the same. Then testosterone kicks in and males develop a penis while the ladies develop a clitoris. So like it or not, the clitoris is a distant relative of your penis. It has its own pleasure-generating nerve endings, it grows when stimulated, and you'd be smart to learn more about it. How much more depends on your lover. Some women prefer vaginal stimulation, but far more prefer both clitoral and vaginal attention. So there's much to be said for exploring her clitoris: touching it directly, rubbing a lubricated finger beside or around it, kissing, sucking. etc. Find out what works best for her—by listening to her words, or moans.

depending on her assertiveness, you'll hear about that—directly or indirectly—sooner or later. Who can blame her? Imagine if she unilaterally declared sex will hence forth involve everything but your penis!

COMING TOGETHER

Why do so many couples strive for simultaneous orgasms? Because they're extraordinary, that's why—especially when they happen spontaneously. There's nothing wrong with going for it, but if you're both focusing on sex as it should be, you're missing sex as it is, and great partnered sex is rooted in the present. This is why many people like the idea of the vaunted "69" position—simultaneous oral sex—for a change of pace, but prefer the one-by-one approach for more regular thrills. You may simply better appreciate what's happening, giving and receiving, when you are concentrating on one or the other. Of course every couple will have to write their own script here, and find what works best for both of them.

If you like to build excitement together, then you may need to lend her a hand. Once we give up the illusion that she should be climaxing from intercourse alone, a world of possibilities opens. Double her pleasure by combining intercourse with manual stimulation.

If you're new to it, don't be surprised if it feels awkward at first. And of course she needs to feel comfortable as well. But once you've blended penis-thrusting with some well-lubricated finger touching and sliding and circling, she may find herself *extremely* comfortable with it. As we saw in *Intercourse*, some positions are better than others for this kind of play. In fact, most other intercourse positions offer better access to the clitoris than does the missionary position, which is the most common. Hmmm, what does that tell us? For one thing, more men need to get on the ball. Or at least try getting off their women.

WHO COMES FIRST?

Generally speaking, it stands to reason (something not totally irrelevant in love and sex) that she should climax before you. Orgasm is a more complicated affair for her. She may need a combination of stimulating input from your fingers, lips, tongue, penis; whatever the two of you have found to work. Let's face it, a man is simple in comparison—give us a photo of a naked woman and a little stroking and—whoops!—we're happy. For her it takes more time.

She's also more likely than you not to shut down after an orgasm. For the most part, when a man comes, he's done. But after she's had her orgasm, she's probably ready for more. And there's little guessing about whether she's sufficiently prepped for you to enter. That makes entry easy for any man who's feeling insecure about his erection. She's ready. She's willing. She's waiting. Feel that situation out and you'll be ready too. Offer her a great sex toy: your penis. Encourage her to hold it and slide it hither and yon. Hey-ho, that feels good! Before you know it, you'll be unfurling the jolly roger and partying with the abandon of pirates.

All in all, there are many reasons for being gallant. Mature. Thoughtful. And they all feel great.

FAKING IT

Most people associate faked orgasms with women. But men do it too, perhaps because a few drinks have dulled their response and they don't want to admit it. Or they just don't want anyone to know they didn't come. But for both men and women there's generally no good reason for this little sexual white lie. It points to a failure of communication. The more important question is, why aren't they capable of talking about expectations and desire? Of course no little fib in itself causes huge problems, but when it happens regularly, not talking about it can make a situation worse. An opportunity for moving closer is squandered, and replaced with increased distance instead of genuine connection.

By the way, if you ever feel the impulse to fake it, you're not alone. One survey revealed that when asked if they ever feel pressured to have an orgasm, close to half of the male respondents said "yes" or "sometimes."[142]

DON'T STOP AT ONE

Men at the frontier of male sexuality are having not one, or even two, but many orgasms in a single, prolonged lovemaking session. Sounds good, right? Where can I sign up, you might be musing. There are two places to begin. One, you can be sixteen with a rock-hard penis and an electric sex drive that has you jerking off every time you sit on the toilet. Or, more realistically for the rest of us, you can investigate spiritual sex.

Sex has been incorporated into sophisticated systems of spiritual growth for hundreds and thousands of years in some traditions around the world. But that doesn't mean you need to learn a foreign language to give it a try. But being open helps: being open to positions other than the missionary position, and being open to the possibility of multiple orgasms.

From our discussion above, we know what the contractile phase of an orgasm is; it's closely related to the expulsion phase—spurting a load of tiny genetic versions of yourself into a vagina or into the world. If we learn to stop stimulating ourselves, whether by intercourse or masturbation, we can halt that transition and stay with the emission phase, during which the prostate gland contracts to empty its fluids in a kind of pre-ejaculatory ejaculation.

As Mantak Chia points out in his book, *The Multi-Orgasmic Man*, sensations accompanying the prostate's contractions can be called "a contractile-phase orgasm."[143] This is where male orgasm begins, and can remain. The effect of this approach leaves wham-bam-thank-you-M'am sex behind and moves it into the stratosphere.

As we move away from the all-too-familiar ejaculation/orgasm, we arrive in a whole new arena of shared sex. Intercourse is prolonged, savored, and mutually satisfying. It's not a matter of trying to get it done fast, or absent-mindedly trying to stretch it out physically. Also, it leads to another area of orgasm unknown to the modern quick-is-good model of sex. Instead of orgasms felt in only our genitals, a bright new possibility looms ahead: whole-body orgasms.

WHOLE-BODY ORGASMS

An orgasm releases all the pressure built-up from your first stirring of desire forward. The more intense the arousal, the more intense the orgasm. So it makes sense to spend enough time with all aspects of lovemaking, including, of course, foreplay, which as we saw in its chapter, is a word, as generally used, in need of expansion.

Chia presents specific techniques in his book to take that built up energy and draw it from your genitals into the rest of your body, including your mind. The result—a whole-body orgasm—is described in different ways. It can be a more diffuse feeling than a genital orgasm, more emotional, and, to get back to where this section began, more spiritual. More on that in *Taoist Sex*.

PENIS

Meet John Thomas. Your manhood, pud, ramrod, or prick.

And welcome to the wonderful world of the penis.

No other part of the male anatomy produces such physical pleasure and such anxiety. A visitor from another planet would marvel at the time and energy spent glorifying, worrying over, fondling and otherwise dwelling on this simple organ. But hey—they wouldn't have grown up with your parents, your peers, Madison Avenue, or Hollywood. Despite what our extraterrestrial friend might think, a penis in the human world is anything but simple. Which he would readily understand if his species featured a two-sex reproductive system.

Let's step back a moment here and look at the penis objectively. What an ingenious solution! Eliminating waste one minute and passing along the precious gift of life the next. Quickly processing millions of impulses to and from the nervous system. Aimlessly idle most of the time, yet able to spring to action at a moment's notice. Decade after decade. Simple? Hardly! That's one impressive unit you have between your legs, mister.

So how do you feel about yours—when you're naked and in the company of at least one other person? Proud, confidant, potent? Or embarrassed. Afraid it's too short. Too long. Too bent, too red, too...whatever.

Like many men, you may not be exactly satisfied with your penis. Why is that? Let's turn to the facts and feelings here. We'll look at penis structure, size, function, fitness, hygiene, and how to guarantee ultimate performance of the most important penis in the world—and you know which that is!

KNOW THYSELF

This may be hard for the great male ego to fathom, but not only is there more to you than your penis; there's more to your genitals too! For the record, here's how the penis fits in.

On the inside, your prostate gland and seminal vesicles produce the non-sperm content of semen. Their fluids lubricate and condition the sperm for its passage through the urethra, or tube, leading to the outside world. On the outside are the testicles and penis.

The glans, or head, has the most nerve endings in your penis. So it's generally the most sensitive part. Uncircumcised males have a foreskin that covers the glans.

The frenulum, also a sensitive, feel-good area, is the area on the underside of your penis where the glans meets the shaft. The shaft doesn't need much explanation. It's the long part, most of a penis's length.

INSIDE OUT

A stiff penis seems deeply rooted because, well, it is. You only see about a third to a half of your penis. It extends inside you and anchors on your pubic bone. It interacts with your inner world as well as the outer one, and is heavily involved with the sometimes shadowy world of thoughts and emotions too. It's fitting, then, that this organ holds the potential to make us more deeply satisfied than any other—it leads us from the outside in, and the inside out, as no other part of us does.

Also, unlike a woman's genitals, which are more contained in her body, you're hanging out there for all the world to see, and judge. And there's no faking it when it comes to action. Either you're hard or you're not.

MEASURING UP

Size. The very word gives many men the willies. Far too many. Convinced their penises are too small, they let their confidence plummet at the very thought. Don't be one of them! Let the facts and figures reassure you. Hey, stand proud!

Most penises range from two to four inches long while soft, and five to six inches hard. Of course those measurements vary greatly depending on whether you just left a warm bed or a cold shower. But what about Tom Twelve-Incher, the porn star? Though some women might like to fantasize about taking him on, most would rather not take a pounding with that kind of tool.

Speaking of women, a vagina's most sensitive area is its outer one-third—the two inches or so that the vast majority of penises easily stimulate. Also, a fit vagina readily adapts to penises of varying shapes and sizes.

Most importantly (to paraphrase Henry Miller), attached to every penis is a man, and the man is what most interests a woman. So stop wishing for something other than what you've got.

Don't spend too much time looking down and judging your penis from above. The perceptual distortion of foreshortening applies; your penis looks smaller than it really is. Check it out in a mirror. Even if you're the rare case of a man with a very small penis, there are many ways to compensate in your lovemaking, and you'll find many of them in this book. Dwell on size and you're just spinning your wheels, fella. Better to pay attention, be present for what an amorous moment is calling for, and get into it!

GET READY, GET SET, GO!

The seduction is over, the breathing is heavy, and you're ready for action. Well, since it's not really happening now, let's take a look inside and see what's happening. Not only is that view interesting, it's helpful. Turns out there's a physiological reason to relax and let it all happen.

You probably know your penis doesn't have a bone. But did you also know it doesn't have any muscle? At least not the kind you normally think of (skeletal muscles like biceps that move bones).

Your penis gets hard when three long chambers in it called corpus cavernosum fill with blood. They're composed of tiny spaces surrounded by smooth muscle tissue, which must relax to let the blood flow in. So even on the microscopic level we see how relaxation is a part of the overall state of sexual excitation.

The inner structure of a penis is perfectly designed for the reproductive function of delivering semen inside a vagina. An erection isn't necessary for that, but the farther inside the semen gets released, the better its chances of fertilizing the awaiting egg.

The various reasons why the erection process might not proceed perfectly are explored in *Impotence*. The good news, however, is that there are many more reasons for textbook erections than otherwise. Even aging, which many men worry about in terms of their sexual ability, is not cause for alarm. Yes, it can slow the whole process down. But women often report more satisfaction because the whole act is more centered in more touch and tenderness than the frantic sexual energy of a throbbing young penis. More wisdom from mother nature.

SPEAKING OF PENISES

No matter what your age, you should be able to talk effectively and unselfconsciously about your penis, with your lover or doctor. In the bedroom, make sure healthy communication is part of the erotic mix. Great sex is reciprocal by nature. Find out her preferences, and tell her yours. If you're uncomfortable or feeling anxious about sex proceeding smoothly, talking can resolve the tension and create more intimacy and connection. It's time to open up, so for starters:

Show-and-Tell Her What Feels Good

Where is your penis most sensitive? What kind of touch turns you on. What kind of stroking? Slapping? Squeezing? Maybe it's obvious to you, but maybe it isn't to her. Don't assume she knows. How could she? Every penis is different. Clue her in. Don't get lost in the fantasy that every lovemaking episode should blaze like the cover of a romance novel! Connection is what counts, the focused fire of mind, body, and emotions. If words are needed, use them. She'll be grateful.

Tell Her How it Works

Every man should know how his penis works, and so should an involved lover. Sexual tension is a wonderful part of the mix, but unspoken desires, assumptions, and feelings can create knots instead of flow. You don't want to kill the mood, just clear the air. So pick an appropriate time—not the peak of passion—to fill her in on the male genital story, which, of course, you have to know in order to tell.

Ask Her to Touch You There

Then move beyond middle school communication. It's amazing how childish and inadequate much of our sexual language is. Maybe someday, when our civilization feels more comfortable with sex as a subject of conversation, we'll have 40 words for sex, like Arctic cultures with their many words for snow. We will have moved past the slang, which has humor and crudeness covered, into genuinely fitting and useful, even beautiful, words for all of sex. Be a pioneer, get ahead of the curve, and create your own sexual language with your lover.

Ask Her to Jerk You Off

Okay, it sounds silly. So find your own words. Mutual masturbation can be great sex play, and highly appropriate for situations where safe sex or avoiding pregnancy is uppermost. It's highly educational too—a perfect way to learn what feels good for both. Let's face it, at a certain point, somebody needs to take charge of the learning curve, and a good candidate is you.

You're a Tough Guy, and So is Your Penis

As you probably know, different kinds of pressures feel good. This is something that might be news to her. Tell her how hard a squeeze, suck, or stroke you can take. Don't expect her to know already.

Tell Her You'd Like a Blow Job

Are those words that work well for you both? If so, great. If not, find some better ones. Make them personal. Make them changeable. Whatever works for you. Going through the ridiculous list of possibilities is a great exercise for breaking the ice. And it will probably demonstrate how helpful humor can be in the bedroom.

TROUBLESHOOTING

Considering its sophisticated and critical role in elimination and sex, your penis is a low-maintenance wonder. Simple hygiene is all that's normally required. Daily washing with soap and water is commonly recommended for an uncircumcised male, to prevent infections or the rarer penile cancer that pro-circumcision arguments often use.

Watch any lesion, red spot, bump, or sore that appears on your penis. If it doesn't go away in a matter of weeks, consult your doctor. Don't be shy. It might not be anything serious, but then again it might be an infection that needs treatment. Worse, and much less often, it can be an early sign of penile cancer which, like most cancers, is much more easily treated when caught early. For other possible problems, see the *Sexually Transmitted Diseases* chapter.

An erection that doesn't disappear is not a laughing matter. Priapism is a potentially dangerous condition that can permanently damage your penis. The veins which normally drain blood from the penis remain blocked. Result? A blood-engorged penis needs attention within 4 hours.[144]

A curved erection signals Peyronie's Disease, a potentially serious problem that can produce a penis too bent or painful for intercourse.[145] For reasons that remain unclear, deposits of plaque appear on the strong membrane called the tunica which encases the interior of a penis. When a penis becomes erect, that deposit doesn't stretch as much as the normal tissue, which causes the curve. Approximately one half of Peyronie's Disease victims impove without treatment; if you don't, and you can't live with the condition, ask your doctor about surgical options, or a new laser treatment that may promise less risk of penis damage.

PORNOGRAPHY

Volcanic desire! Horny housewives! Smut-crazed sluts in heat! Yes! Yes! Yes!

And in this corner, stern-faced moralists and your own inner judge shouting No! No! No!

Porno sure gets the blood moving—both in those pumping up their sexual energy and those getting red in the face over its alleged negative impact on society.

So what's the verdict? Depends on the case in point. The word "pornography" gets applied to everything from a sanitized Playboy photo to debased XXX child-porn videos to discreet literary erotica.

Many would make the case that pornography encourages violence toward, or at least degradation of, women by a male-dominated industry; others counter that it actually reduces rape by providing a private sexual outlet for those who would otherwise act out their frustration in the world.

Healthy sex involves consenting participants. That excludes any kind of coercion, or use of minors by adults. But it includes many forms of sexual expression and enjoyment deemed unacceptable by some. And there's the rub, as it were. Throughout history and around the world, art or writing deemed pleasantly arousing to one person has been judged blatantly obscene by another. In many cases the latter has suppressed the offending work and punished those involved in its production.

A BRIEF HISTORY OF THE FORBIDDEN

The contemporary legal definition of pornography applies to a work that an "average person" using "contemporary community standards" finds basically "prurient" and lacking "serious literary, artistic, political, or scientific value."[146] That's vague enough. But look up "prurient" in the dictionary and you'll find that it refers to an "inordinate" interest in sex. And "inordinate" means exceeding ordinary limits. It begins to sound like a word puzzle. But of course it's not a game because pornography and its effects are a serious matter for society. We'll leave the legal fine points to the lawyers, and look briefly at the history of the subject.

Pornography derives from a Greek word referring to art or writing about prostitutes, implying an erotic and/or arousing quality. Since classical days there has been a running battle about the nature of acceptable sexually-oriented material. It's interesting to note how societal changes have changed the face of pornography.

For example, consider how different attitudes were when most people lived in close contact with farm animals and their natural sexuality, or when classes of women were considered too delicate for much but motherly duties (and not to have much in the way of sexual feelings).[147]

As you look at examples in Western history—from the Bible's *Song of Songs* to John Cleland's eighteenth-century *Fanny Hill* to James Joyce's *Ulysses* in our own century—you see examples of work once outlawed as obscene and later redeemed, sold, and read freely.

It's only been a couple of hundred years since printed material of any kind became readily available, and only since the post-war period in our country when sexual material in particular has been widely available. Then the Sexual Revolution thirty years ago intensified the debate considerably. Now the popularity of the Internet has rekindled it again, and, as always, it's fueled by changing attitudes to sexuality in general.

Since society as a whole can't easily decide what's acceptable, no wonder men can feel conflicted about using and enjoying pornography.

TAKING THE MATTER IN HAND

Maybe you found a hidden stash of pornographic movies in a closet at home, or discovered a racy magazine in the trash at school. Whatever your introduction to pornography, there was probably a shady element to the discovery. That's of course understandable in an environment of little if any communication about sexuality.

But what was clear, if troubling, was how it made you feel. In short, it turned you on. Add the newly discovered act of masturbation, and the link was solidified. In fact, much of the historical debate about porn has gone hand in hand with the debate about masturbation. Consider the opinion of the famous theologian St. Thomas Aquinas, who felt that masturbation was second only to homicide in the hierarchy of sins—an intense judgment against self-pleasuring if ever there was one! So pornography was linked with deep-seated views about masturbation's wasting semen, debilitating boys and men, and generally harming society's ability to prosper. And while masturbation is a difficult activity to control directly, the next best option was controlling the material presumably encouraging it, which, of course, was pornography.

As we'll see in *Taoist Sex*, indiscriminate masturbation is still considered by some (in addition to those with traditionally anti-sex beliefs) to have less than positive effects. But today it's much easier to find those for whom pornography does in fact have redeeming value, for individuals and for society as a whole.

LISTENING TO WOMEN

So men historically have had, and continue to have, opposing judgments about pornography, as increasingly do women. Probably the most common complaint is that women find most pornography geared to men's sexual fantasies, and they simply don't find it arousing. The sight of an actress licking and rubbing her nipples is not universally appreciated, to say the least.

With radical feminists, the judgments are more severe. They see insults at best and incitement to rape at worst. Men should consider their arguments. For instance, imagine how it would feel to know that a physically stronger gender was watching movies depicting naked men being physically assaulted, say stomped in a bathtub until the water ran red. What men would cheer that image? And is it unreasonable to consider whether less explicit movies contain some of that general tone? Since men don't exist in a vacuum, they should try to see pornography through the eyes of women. Just like communication of any kind, it's a two-way street. One subject that should be discussed is the association of pornography with rape. Though on a societal level alleged incidents of actresses being forced into sex on camera have been largely discredited, men should look within themselves for the final ramification of this issue. Sexual coercion is always wrong, no matter who's doing and who's receiving.

Porn For Both of You

Needless to say, pornography is not universally condemned by women. In fact, by one estimate women bring home one quarter of rented X-rated videos.[148] What's more, women are making more of them too. The most well-known example is the work of Candida Royalle and her company, Femme Productions. Her stated intent is to create erotic films both men and women will enjoy. To her credit, unless the actors involved are lovers in real life, they use condoms. Her website (www.royale.com) notes that she is the only maker of adult films to be a member of the American Association of Sex Educators, Counselors, and Therapists.

COMPARING PROS AND CONS

With so much historical criticism of pornography, is there anything positive left to say about it? Well sure. After all, something draws millions of men and women to it in all its heterosexual, gay, or lesbian forms. It increases sexual arousal. It enhances pleasure. It *feels good.*

For many individuals, sexuality is a domain of discomfort. They just don't know much about it. Pornography can broaden their sexual horizons. They can learn techniques safely and legally in the privacy of their own home. Some couples combine it with mutual stimulation. They use it to encourage sexual communication. For many men and women, it arouses their sexual fantasies, and provides a sexual outlet when none other exist, or when a relationship fails to do so. Sex therapists often recommend it to jump-start sexual desire.

Besides the issues of female degradation discussed earlier, some experts caution against using pornography as a model of sexual behavior in the real world. Since much hard-core pornography focuses on close-up shots of genitals, it's a far cry from the new sexual model which puts a woman's real needs on equal footing with those of a man. Foreplay, for instance, should be viewed as taking more than a token few moments for either party.

Another unrealistic aspect of many pornographic films are huge penises and instant erections. If men try to measure their own penises and responses by those standards, their own self-confidence could suffer. Sex viewed without any emotional component other than lust is fine in the fantasy world, but problematic in the real one.

Kept in perspective, reading about or viewing adult actors engaged in consenting sex has a legitimate place in the lives of many men and women, who pay the multibillion dollar profits that will move the industry into the future full steam ahead.

GETTING INTO PORNOGRAPHY

It's hard to imagine that fifty years ago it wasn't easy to find erotic materials. Now with commercial phone sex and the Internet, you don't even have to leave home. So what's out there in the universe of porn? Here's a quick survey of three main areas today: books and magazines, videos, and online pornography.

Books and Magazines

Since the word "pornography" has such an unsavory feeling about it, "erotica" has appeared as a more tasteful alternative. With its softcore sound (similar to Beethoven's sixth symphony), erotica is largely associated with literary or fine art erotic materials. You have many genres to choose from, representing all sexual orientations. Collections of female fantasies are now joined by Bob Berkowitz's male fantasy collection, *His Secret Life*. Older, historical fiction ranges from classics like Ovid to D.H. Lawrence and Henry Miller and Anaïs Nin. Note that reading porn written by women can work just fine for men. The big bookstores don't stock a lot of small press porn. Try smaller bookstores or online booksellers. Porn books on tape add spice to that long car ride or view from the mountaintop at sunset.

Magazines run the gamut and add the power of pictures. The famous soft porn world of *Playboy* introduced the Sexual Revolution to millions. Now the magazine rack offers raunchier offerings and a ton of 900 number ads to make the experience interactive. Whatever your sexual interest you can find a relatively inexpensive magazine to match it.

Videos

Between cable television and the neighborhood video store, men now have easy access to a virtual flood of pornography. Most of it is far from Hollywood production quality, but that's not the primary source of gratification here. As mentioned earlier, women producers have added a new aspect of believable story lines and videos more likely to appeal to you and her. Explicitly educational videos advertised everywhere can in fact be educational and a turn-on too.

Then there's the option of making your own. The price of video cameras has dropped dramatically, but if you still can't justify the expense, rent one for a day. Then you can play your own music for a soundtrack, arrange the lighting that you think will work best, and...action!...you're ready. Making love on camera is a fantasy many men and women respond to in a big way. Obviously you'll want to be careful where you store the resulting tape; you don't want it finding its way onto the Internet!

Online Porn

First-time computer users will be amazed at what already exists in cyberspace. Most major magazines and video companies have websites offering all manner of pictures, video, and audio erotica. On another portion of the phone lines, bulletin boards offer household-to-household discussions without the graphics of the World Wide Web. On either venue, discussions are frank and personal, and are intense, but just the latest examples of pornography offering sexual excitement, for better or worse, without guilt, shame, risk, emotional involvement. Like the rest of the Internet, the sheer amount of information in the area of sex is staggering; you can find catalogs, performance schedules, news, pornographic pictures and videos, frequently asked questions, and just about anything else you desire.

PROSTATE

You wake up in the dark with an urge to urinate. Damn! Third time tonight. Okay, same drill: trudge off to the bathroom and stand for a minute before dribbling a weak stream into the toilet.

Welcome to midlife. As if graying hair and an expanding waistline weren't enough, here comes a new hassle. But this symptom is announcing more than just the passage of time. This symptom you need to do something about, starting with a visit to your doctor. You might very well be fine, but it's definitely time to find out for sure.

Let's cut to the chase: ignoring prostate gland symptoms can lead to impotence, incontinence, and death. 42,000 American men die from prostate cancer every year. It's second only to lung cancer as a cause of death for men. Of course, the picture isn't totally bleak. The majority of prostate problems aren't cancerous, and you can take steps now to point you in the direction of good prostate health and long-term sexual fitness.

LISTEN TO YOUR WAKE-UP CALL

According to the National Cancer Society, prostate cancer is now twice as common as lung cancer in American men. If you think it's just a disease for old men, think again. Frank Zappa died of it at 52. Fortunately, there are others, like General Norman Schwarzkopf, who have gone public with their problems with, and victories over, prostate cancer.

Other celebrity cases have brought prostate problems into the limelight. Methods of diagnosis and treatment have improved, and effective preventative steps enable you to prevent and even reverse early symptoms.

This is good news for any man who values his sex life.

MEET YOUR PROSTATE GLAND

If you're like most American men, you don't know much about your prostate. For your continued sexual fitness, however, the time to learn more is right now.

The prostate, a walnut-sized gland beneath your bladder and above your rectum, works in your body's reproduction department. In general, glands secrete substances, and the prostate's secretion contributes to the mix called semen. About a third of total semen volume is the prostate's thin and milky lubricating fluid, which nourishes the sperm while helping it travel up and out of your penis.

Apart from its reproductive function, the prostate can also affect urination. A tube called the urethra, which connects the bladder with the end of the penis, runs through the middle of the prostate gland. When the prostrate swells for any reason, it can pinch the urethra, restricting the flow of urine and creating symptoms like weak or frequent urination, and pain and soreness anywhere in the genitourinary tract or surrounding area.

The following symptoms indicate that it's time to ask your doctor for a prostate exam:
- The feeling that you haven't emptied your bladder after urinating
- The need to urinate several times during one night (nocturnia)
- A weak urine stream, or stopping and starting repeatedly during urination
- The urge to urinate soon after having done so
- Problems starting a urine stream
- The inability to postpone urination

TYPES OF PROSTATE PROBLEMS

American men are more likely to see a doctor for prostate symptoms than for any other health problem.[149] Those symptoms signal one of three conditions: Benign Prostatic Hyperplasia, Prostatitis, or Prostate Cancer.

Benign Prostatic Hyperplasia (BPH) is not cancer, though it results from prostate cells growing abnormally. Here the gland expands with a nonmalignant tumor, constricting the urethra and causing difficulties with urine flow.

BPH doesn't spread through the body as cancer can. It can be treated successfully, and in many cases, easily. Treatment depends on the severity of the symptoms. Many physicians adopt a "wait and see" approach. The next step might be drugs to reduce the swelling. Herbal remedies are also available and are becoming increasingly popular. If symptoms progress, several surgical procedures are available either to enlarge the urethra or reduce the size of the prostate.

Prostatitis also results in prostate swelling, but is usually caused by a bacterial infection. Pain is more likely than in BPH in the penis, in the rectum, or in ejaculation. Antibiotics are the usual treatment. Prostatitis can also result from prostatic fluid backing up for reasons other than infection. In this case a physician may simply recommend more frequent ejaculation. Nonbacterial prostatitis is more of an unknown. Warm sitz baths are often recommended.

Prostate cancer is the most serious of these conditions. 20% of men seeking help with prostate symptoms will receive this diagnosis. As with other cancers, *early detection significantly boosts the odds of recovery.* When prostate cancer spreads to other parts of the body, especially to bone marrow, the prognosis is poor. Surgery for prostate cancer carries the risk of severing nerves involved with erection and ejaculation; impotence and incontinence can result. However, recent advances in those procedures offer better results, and even better surgery and therapies are on the horizon.

DETERMINE YOUR RISK

Who's at greatest risk for prostate problems? The two biggest factors are race and family history. For reasons currently unknown, African Americans are at greatest risk, Japanese-Americans are on the lower end of the scale, with Caucasians and Latinos in between.

Having a family history of prostate problems also elevates your risk. Men with fathers, uncles, or brothers who had prostate cancer should start the standard prostate tests earlier than others.

Some studies have suggested a link between prostate cancer and vasectomies, especially after 20 years, but most doctors dispute those studies.

SMILE AND BEND OVER FOR THE DOCTOR

By age fifty—or forty if you're considered higher risk—you should be having prostate checks as part of your annual physical examinations. The tests are simple.

The Digital Rectal Examination (DRE) is the first and simplest way to gauge the prostate's health. The test consists of a doctor donning a thin glove, lubricating a finger, inserting it in the anus, and feeling your prostate gland. He will easily be able to judge its size. There is no physical pain or discomfort in the procedure, though some men are embarrassed by pleasurable sensations or even an erection if nerves extending into the penis are stimulated.

Though a good way to check for prostate swelling, a DRE is not a sure test for cancer. Some tumors might be positioned where they can't be felt, or are too small to feel at all, so another test was developed which doesn't rely on mere touching. Called the Prostate-Specific Antigen test, or PSA, it's a blood test which measures antigens produced only in the prostate, and produced at higher levels with prostate swelling. An ultrasound or biopsy will likely be the next step for those whose tests produce high levels. The tricky part is what to do after that, because there is no medical consensus on how or when to treat prostate cancer.

Some cancers are more aggressive than others. If a tumor is small, dormant, or slow-growing, a doctor may simply advise a "watchful waiting" strategy. Older patients may choose this strategy rather than surgery or radiation therapy with potentially unacceptable impact on their quality of life, such as impotence and incontinence. Younger men have the same decision to make if the cancer is small and contained in the prostate.

Several herbal, drug, hormone, and surgical options are available to treat prostate problems from the least to most severe. For men with no symptoms other than anxiety about the future of their prostate, there are proactive actions to take now for optimum prostate health.

TWELVE TIPS FOR A HEALTHY PROSTATE

Include a Prostate Exam in Your Annual Physical

If you're forty or older, your annual physical should include a rectal exam. After fifty (or forty for high-risk men) have a PSA done too. If your doctor doesn't include these tests, ask why not. Remember, the sooner you're aware of prostate problems, the easier they are to treat.

Eat Less Red Meat

...and other high fat foods. High-fat-eating can increase the production of testosterone, which has been identified as a factor in prostate enlargement.

Enjoy Cooked Tomatoes

They were highlighted in a 1995 study by the National Institute of Cancer. Dishes such as pizza and spaghetti were found to significantly reduce the incidence of prostate cancer. An antioxidant called lycopene, abundant in cooked tomatoes, may be the reason. The findings confirm other research revealing a low incidence of prostate problems in the Mediterranean region where tomato products are prevalent.

Include Soy Products in Your Diet

New research points to their ability to prevent prostate cancer. Tofu, soy juice, miso, and tempeh are all good examples.

Make Sure You Get Enough Zinc

The mineral associated with some reputed aphrodisiacs is also thought to ward off prostate cancer, probably because it boosts overall immune system strength.

Drink Plenty of Water

An insufficient supply of water weakens the prostate. Water makes a great substitute for coffee, which can irritate the prostate.

Drink Green Tea

Researchers at Mayo Clinic have identified an anti-tumor substance in green tea that they think may be responsible for the lower incidence of prostate cancer in the Far East, where green tea is the beverage of choice.[148] They are currently running tests to isolate the cancer-preventing phytochemicals.

Try Herbs and Vitamins

Thousands of men have discovered herbal or traditional medicine through the use of prostate-friendly saw palmetto. A small palm tree native to southeastern Florida, its berries in pill or extract form can reduce an enlarged prostate and contribute to its health. Also recommended are pumpkin seeds and licorice (which shouldn't be taken in large quantities).

Vitamins associated with prostate health are vitamin E, vitamin C, selenium, and vitamins A and D. As with the mineral zinc, these vitamins should be taken in controlled doses. Talk with your doctor or a nutritionist for the proper regimen for you.

Exercise

If you need motivation to exercise as you know you should, consider its benefits for your prostate gland. Aerobic exercise has been shown in many instances to strengthen your immune system. Since it's commonly recognized that cancer cells exist in many more prostates than those exhibiting the developed disease, some speculate that exercise is one of the factors which keep them at bay. Men with prostate symptoms should consider curtailing activities like bike or horseback riding, which put stress on the whole genitourinary tract, or ask a bike shop about new split seats designed to minimize that problem.

Manage Your Stress

Oriental medicine teaches us that a flow of energy within us called chi (or ki) is responsible for our health and happiness. Prostate symptoms are sufficient reason for some men to take the philosophy seriously. Stress is one factor that disrupts a healthy flow of energy. Meditation, exercise, and positive thinking are all excellent ways to restore balance. Getting in touch with negative emotions is also helpful. And relaxation can be powerful medicine. There are many more ways to combat stress—such as sex itself—which are explored elsewhere in this book.

Have Sufficient Orgasms

Now there's one prescription that's easy to accept. Since the prostate gland continuously creates fluid for semen, there are indications that too few orgasms may contribute to a backup of prostatic fluid and result in complications such as prostatitis. Some research suggests frequent orgasm as part of the cure; others dispute that. The general consensus points to not too many orgasms, but not too few either. Again, an individual assessment is needed, perhaps in concert with a trusted doctor, based on individual criteria.

Do Your Kegels

Exercises that strengthen and tone your pelvic floor, or pubococcygeus (PC), muscles are good for your prostate gland. Not only can they boost your sexual pleasure, but they can help keep a prostate from enlarging. Look for details in *Kegels*.

SEDUCTION

Your eyes meet. Time slows. You feel a connection and sense an opening. Maybe you step into it or maybe you don't. Maybe you're married, or she's engaged, or any number of barriers intervene. But for a moment you bask in the charged potential of what may be, or at least what might have been.

It can happen at a party, in a business meeting, or anywhere at all. It's a surprise, a moment brimming with energy and potential and a surge of excitement. If circumstances allow, words follow. Then a casual touch. Maybe a kiss. And after that, who knows? The vast realm of sexuality opens before you.

When your eyes meet hers for the millionth time, over breakfast or in a car with kids bouncing in the back seat, the call for seduction still rises above the day-to-day. Different tactics might be needed, but the end goal of a romp in naked passion remains the same.

Seduction is a flow from eye contact to flirting to dating to all the scents and tastes and touches which gradually become, in the best case scenario, indistinguishable from sexual arousal. In one sense, the best seduction is itself foreplay. Especially if foreplay is considered less a contained unit of sex than an attitude of openness, expansiveness, and play of intimacy.

Flirting and seduction are more a province of attitudes and emotions than physical fitness. But grooming figures in big time, because how you look not only advertises who you are, it can tell a woman much about what to expect. In fact, as scientists look seriously at flirtation and seduction, they offer some surprising conclusions about why we do the flirtatious things we do, and how directly they relate to behavior of birds and bugs and bears.

PICK YOUR APPROACH

Mention the word "seduction" to a woman and you might get a cold shoulder. After all, it has a somewhat deflated history of manipulation and lies and other underhanded male efforts to get a woman into bed, after which, to her chagrin and anger, her knight without shining armor would collect his underwear and shoes and sneak out the door.

But that's not what seduction needs to be, or should be. We should expect others to treat us the way we treat them. Nonetheless, there is an intention involved, an effort to get something going.

The *Fit For Sex* approach goes beyond manipulation. Here's a better way to define sexual seduction: *initiating and guiding efforts to get a woman to join you in mutually satisfying sex.* There—no one needs to be annoyed with that approach. In fact, it's a win-win situation. Forget cajoling until you're blue in the face, or turning red with anger when your net gain in the sex column again comes up zero. Instead, you get what you want and so does she.

Ultimately it's a black and white choice. Either you're focused on what *you* want, or you're proceeding according to what *both of you* want.

SEDUCING AND MARKETING

Pairing seduction with marketing might turn off some (okay—many) men and women. But there's a very good reason for doing so. By way of explanation, let's talk cars.

Remember when Detroit was selling poor-quality cars? The unspoken formula was to go with their planning, producing, and selling for maximum profit and the customer be damned! The annoying problem was that their buyers were deserting in droves. No amount of fancy advertising could hide the fact that the cars didn't measure up against new competition that dared to offer quality. What changed? Detroit started listening to its customers, who preferred not to have knobs come off in their hands and resale value plummet after a year and a half.

Marketing at its best listens to what consumers want and need, and provides it.

Does this relate to getting Betty into the sack? You bet! If your seduction resembles car sales techniques from 1963, why should you expect her to swoon tonight? The point is, look at it from her point of view. That's fine seduction for the new millennium, and that's the way to get where you want to go.

You want her. Okay, now get her to want you too!

How to start? Look at it this way. In a very short time she will size up the who, why, where, when, and how of you and your intentions. So each of those has to feel right to her. They should feel right to you too.

WHO AND WHY

The essential first step in seduction is having someone to seduce. And while that sounds obvious, it introduces an important point: *who* is the object of your desire?

Preceding even that is the foundation of the whole enterprise: what do you want? That's the *why* of seduction. The *who* and the *why* are intimately connected, and very much determine the look and feel of your seduction.

A wild night in a new bedroom? A soul mate with whom to traverse life's peaks and valleys? An enlivened interlude with your mate of twenty years? If you like strip clubs, look for a woman who gets off watching hunks dancing without shirts. If you like Sartre, find someone able to enjoy a good depression at the beach.

Just keep in mind, as Henry Miller reminds us, that attached to every vulva is a woman.[151] If you're looking only for a vulva, why not try one of those genitally-correct inflatable dolls? But if you're man enough to engage the whole of a woman, well then, the game's afoot!

You're looking for a woman who looks great, cooks great, has a great job and/or is great with kids, and is great in bed. Or are you? Maybe you're just looking for a good time, and someone who is looking for the same. A fling. Of course you'll prefer not for her to be thinking short-term if you're thinking long.

Who are you? What are you looking for? Make sure you have at least rough answers to those questions to aid the seduction; you'll avoid hardships later.

Of course you can't know everything in advance. Some questions get answered along the way. So now it's time to stop pondering the fine points and actually get up and get out there. It's time for the *where* of seduction.

WHERE AND WHEN

The good news is that there are millions of women out there looking for men. The tricky part is finding one who shares your interests and also turns you on. You can leave it to chance, if that works for you, or you could put some planning into it. Different places have pros and cons, which should be considered before jumping in with both feet.

Bars.   Happy hour! Dirty dancing! Get down! The scene's great for letting your hair down, but maybe not so great if you don't have much of it left. Also, it's probably not the place to find the intellectual type. But you never know! If you're unsure, try it. You might like it!

Personal ads.   The accent is on the personal-ized; the advantage is sending out feelers in areas of real interest. Worth a try as long as you're sure it's worth the money. So is the latest variation: the Internet. Find a cyber-pen-pal and see what develops. The initial impersonal aspect of writing allows you to ask specific questions. Just find a way to inquire about looks that doesn't sound like you are inspecting livestock, or leave it to a photo request.

At work. Could be trouble! Big trouble. Remember, if the initial heat cools, you'll still be passing in the hallway, or sitting across the table from her in meetings. So spend more time up front making sure the attraction is coming from some other place than only your trousers. If not, pass this one up and save yourself some big regrets.

Clubs or volunteer organizations. Several advantages here. You avoid the blind date fiascoes by spending some time observing before stepping up and making your intentions known. Some major interest or value is already shared in being a member of the organization, and you're not home moaning about being at home. So definitely, get out there. Get involved. Broaden your horizons, whether or not you come home with a broad (and you probably won't if you use that word).

Word of mouth. Reliable but not foolproof. Friends of friends can be good—someone has some reason for pairing you. Find out why! And go for the occasional blind date. Open yourself to the whims of fate. Maybe a group activity with the friends in question will be less stressful and more fun.

Open your eyes. Any place can be the right place. Think positive and send forth the right vibes. Who knows who will pick them up? When your mind and senses are open—that's seduction's most important *when*. Whether you're in the laundromat or in your shared kitchen, when you feel an openness and you think she does or can, there you go. Then you're ready for the *how* of seduction.

EIGHT TIPS FOR SUPERCHARGING SEDUCTION

One of the most common mistakes of seduction is getting lost in technique. Remember, she wants to know who you are. Most likely she's interested in a relationship of whatever duration. Sure, there are a few classic pointers to keep in mind, but be yourself. Find out what makes her tick, what makes her feel good. But most of all, don't forget to enjoy yourself—never underestimate the power of a heartfelt smile!

Use the Power of Grooming

You don't have to smell like soap, but no one gets off on sour body odor. If you like scents, try a cologne, but keep it light; you won't impress her if she feels like showering after you've touched her. Being clean and stylish go a long way. Choose fashion, hair styles, glasses, etc. that match your body and face type. If you're unsure what that is, don't be afraid to ask a hair stylist or salesperson where you buy your clothes.

Get Serious about Eye Contact

Catching her eye can be the glorious start of it all. But be careful that it's not the end of it just as fast. Prime eye contact can too easily turn into discomfort and retreat if extended too long. Cool it! You can always return for more! She may read a stare as overly aggressive, especially if mixed with overt stares at her chest or rear end.

She'd prefer to be appreciated in subtler ways. Scope out her jewelry or hair and then flick your eyes to and from the delights below. Notice how she dresses and makes herself up. She'll welcome sincere comments about those things, which you can't notice when fixing a leaden stare between her legs.

Later, women appreciate eye contact when talking. True, the Navaho consider that rude, but most women expect it. If eyes are indeed the window to the soul, and if she's interested in you, she'll want you looking in.

Create an Opening with Body Language

It's an art, not a science. So don't sweat the details. Just remember the basics: keep your shoulders back to reflect that confidence that's in you somewhere. Lean slightly forward (to place that tantalizing touch), and avoid barricading yourself behind crossed arms or legs. Remember, it's openness you'd like to project, not in-her-face come-and-get-me.

Don't Lose Her when You Open Your Mouth

What are the sure-to-get-you-in, most foolproof pick-up lines of all time? There are none. Each woman and each setting is different. And every "haven't-I-seen-you-here-before" sleeper inwardly moves her back ten steps. What you want is for her to feel good, emotionally and physically. Try to find out who she is and what she wants. In short, let things develop naturally.

A classic sales technique is not asking questions that can be answered with a "yes" or "no." Instead, ask her how she feels or what she thinks about something. Get her talking. Find out who she is. Then you'll move quickly past the artificial openers.

Hold off on the latest joke you just heard at work. Unless you're lucky, you'll be left slapping your knee and guffawing while she scans the room for the nearest exit.

Go Slow

This applies to most every aspect of seduction. Make your first touches easy and natural, even if their placement has a slight edge to it. A light touch on her shoulder or the small of her back is better than grabbing her hand too soon. The same goes for kissing. Start easy. Be exploratory. And don't be so anxious to talk that you smother quiet moments to absorb what's been said. You'll know when to speed up. If you're paying attention, you'll pick up unmistakable signals.

Wine and Dine

A candlelit table in a dark restaurant. Two chairs on a balcony over water. Many classic seduction images hold their power for good reason: they work. Use your setting to increase her feel-good movement in your direction. Make the little extra efforts that mean a lot to a woman. Order flowers after the first, or latest, date. Leave provocative voice mail. Open the door for her. Make her a meal. When you make her feel special, which hopefully you truly feel, then good things happen.

Be Honest

There's always an impulse to say whatever works, to embellish the facts to your advantage, and to just plain lie about something you wish were different. Forget it. Whatever short-term gain you enjoy will be demolished in the long run. When you prove you can't be trusted, no slick moves or fancy words will regain what you've lost. Stick with the facts. Trust the truth.

Overcome Rejection

Unless you're a surefire combination of Leonardo DiCaprio and Harrison Ford, your best seduction efforts will at some point end with rejection. No problem! It's just good old-fashioned feedback, telling you what you're doing right and what you're doing wrong. In fact, that's how you learn. Is it one type of woman you're having trouble with? Maybe she's not for you. One move that's not working with your wife anymore? Maybe you need something new.

Seduction, like life, never stays the same. Everything changes. It'd be pretty dull otherwise. Accept that, and keep refining your style.

SEX APPEAL

Sam says he doesn't care about it—yet he's a sharp dresser and tends to push his chest out around women. So he may not consciously think about sex appeal, but it's definitely important to him—and to most other men who don't live in a monastery.

The whole subject can sound trivial. But nonetheless it's a strong vibe, coming from deep within. Hey, those are your genes talking when you consider what to say, how to move, and what to wear around your wife, girlfriend, or the new woman at work.

So exactly what is it? Well, typically it flows from power. Intelligence. Self-confidence. And good looks. Yet those are just part of the initial sexual impression you make on a woman.

We'll look at several character traits and see how they fit together to form sex appeal. And to illustrate we'll look at how they play in Hollywood.

SEX APPEAL, TAKE...ONE

You're handsome, tough, suave, and sexy.

And you're lucky, because not everyone compares so favorably with Sean Connery.

But what about the real you? Would you call yourself smooth? Sexy? Who defines these things anyway? Well, Hollywood certainly does in part. Sure, we go to the movies to be thrilled, amused, and inspired. But we also go to see the stars. In their cinematic roles, actors become more than mere humans; they become ideals of looks and behavior and values.

We also see films to see new possibilities; somewhere amid the moving pictures and sounds, we can acquire new attitudes. Hollywood long ago realized the power of sex, and for decades our sexual self-image has slowly been modified by the art form called movies.

And have you noticed how your own preferences for male actors has changed over time? Actors change. You change. But the importance of image and personal magnetism remains constant.

Here then is a brief survey and primer on how to nourish your sex appeal, with examples of actors who radiate it. The point, as we'll see, is not to mimic them, but ultimately to deliver a command performance as yourself.

HOW TO BOOST YOUR SEX APPEAL

Be Sexy

Sounds easy. So what's the key? Well, appearance matters, but that's not the essence of sex appeal. Remember, when silent films became talkies, some of the biggest stars faded fast because once they opened their mouths the thrill was gone.

For birds it's easy: display colorful feathers or do a special dance. For men, attracting a prospective sexual partner can be more complicated. The bottom line is this: sex appeal flows from how we feel, not just how we look.

Take Sean Connery. Mr. Masculinity. Even a tough movie critic like Pauline Kael loved to watch him. Why? Well, most people would agree he's handsome, and strong (he was once Scotland's entry competing for the title of Mr. Universe). The Scottish accent certainly doesn't hurt. But the guy exudes self-confidence, especially in the role that quickly became a parody of itself, James Bond. Even in dire straits, 007 was always comfortable being himself, self-esteem never an issue. Surely that was a major part of his sexual vibe, and explains the huge influence of the character at the time.

Confidence flows from positive self-esteem. Attracting someone is easier when you feel attractive (but not full of yourself). If you feel low self-esteem, you can change that. Think about what your strengths are and start by concentrating on them. It's easy to change your appearance, so start there, gradually dressing with more authority and style. Practice asking for what you want. For further techniques along those lines, see the chapter on *Seduction*.

Do you wish you had someone else's hair? Someone else's penis? Those are great examples of torpedoing your self-esteem. In a recent survey, women were asked to rate male qualities they find most attractive, and the winner wasn't a man's looks. What took the honors was personality.[152] What matters most to most women is who you are on the inside.

Brad Pitt, Tom Cruise—they certainly have the looks, but will they prove themselves over time to have what it takes on the inside? For them, time will tell, but it has already told us about Sean Connery and the durability of his attraction. He made the difficult leap out of the spy business and played a range of characters with equal success. Most of them exude sex appeal. So can you. Here are a few other ways to get there.

Be Cool

Every generation defines cool anew. But one of Hollywood's all-time coolest was Steve McQueen. Whether playing a cowboy on TV, a San Francisco cop, or an escaped war prisoner on a motorcycle, he was often the loner, but always Mr. Cool.

In times when more and more men have female bosses, or earn less than their sexual partners, perhaps a little detachment is not a bad thing. A little distance. Men need to stand back and think on things. Regroup. Preserve their dignity. McQueen shows us how. His emotions were understated. A squint here, an icy stare there. But you always knew the wheels were turning inside. Can a loner be passionate? He certainly could. You saw it when a smile lit that face from within.

The clothes helped. Not being much for conformity, Steve McQueen wasn't often in a suit. Given his childhood brushes with the law, his outsider persona wasn't an act. The jean thing was his natural style, at a time when it wasn't the establishment's.

His body, or more to the point, his physical presence was cool too. He lifted weights, but not to advertise his body. There was power in his walk, without the John Wayne swagger. Again, an understated presence.

More and more men today are going for washboard abs and the chiseled chest look. That's cool, but as an end in itself? Women are drawn less to muscle than men commonly believe. In other words, physical fitness is good, but women like a body with a light on upstairs.

We don't need to be like Steve in every way, but we can sure learn from his cool.

Be Tough

Then there's the other famous San Francisco cop, also a renegade, also a loner. But Dirty Harry was different. And so is Clint Eastwood. He is taller than McQueen, and used even fewer words. In the spaghetti- westerns his silence was monumental. On the other end of his career, in the western that finally won him an Academy Award, he still was very tall, very dark and handsome—and very silent.

In that silence is power. Dirty Harry's .44 magnum was certainly powerful. But the image of the cop behind it made it more so. Tough took on a new look.

But is tough sexy? Certainly not to the women who were turned off by Dirty Harry. But the interesting thing about Clint's toughness is how it matured with time. This is a great lesson from Hollywood. The roles change in an actor's career. And if he stays in touch, so does the actor himself. Suddenly Clint's a wandering photographer in the Midwest wooing Meryl Streep. Still a loner, still toughing out what life sets before him, but no longer swinging at it with his fists. In fact, now he's downright sensitive. Strong. With sex appeal to spare.

Be Sensitive

He spent half his career playing thugs in second-rate movies and then emerged with a heart of gold in arguably the greatest love story ever filmed. The actor was Humphrey Bogart, and the movie is *Casablanca*.

Somehow ol' dogfaced Bogie rose to the top. How times change. Today he would probably never be more than a character actor, and certainly not a sex symbol in a white dinner jacket. But there again, it wasn't just the look. The power came from within.

When the movie opens, Rick is as hard-boiled as they come. Looking out for number one. But then his long-lost lover walks into his cafe. Sam plays *As Time Goes By* and Bogie begins the long journey back to the present. By the time the plane's engine sputters to life on the foggy runway, the circle is complete. Love prevails. The tough guy proves what he's really made of inside. Pure gold.

Bogie swept Ingrid Bergman away because of who he was, not how he looked. In the end he did the right thing. For her. For her husband. And for him. What a guy. Take a cue from Bogart. Be as tough as you like, but keep your heart open.

Be Good-Looking

One of the best examples of a durable male sex symbol in Hollywood is Robert Redford. Once again we see that his power is more than skin deep. Whether a reporter, baseball player or prison warden, he stands for something. But of course there's no denying his good looks. Give him credit for always trying to move beyond that—he took his gift and built something real with it.

However much or little you resemble Redford or Leonardo DiCaprio or Denzel Washington isn't really important. Every man has something going for him in the looks department, and you can boost your sex appeal by making the most of your personal strengths.

Grooming is square one. Even a cowboy coming off the range for a Saturday night starts with a bath. Without cleanliness you won't get to first base. Fresh breath, clean teeth, etc.—these are the basics upon which your chances for success begin.

Why not make an effort to see what fashion styles are in, and how they relate to your body? Are pleated pants right for you? Ask a female friend how you look and what might make you look better. If you wear glasses, do they complement your face?

Are your fingernails clean? Beard trimmed? Sure, they're little things, but not to a woman. There are many ways to make your looks work for you, not against you. There's nothing artificial about that. You're just making it easier for her to see your strengths.

Be Expressive

If life were like *A Streetcar Named Desire*, it would be intolerably exhausting. Marlon Brando's performance as Stanley Kowalski in that 1951 film put method acting on center stage. It was felt, not faked. He went down into his emotions and came up with the raw intensity that would eventually lead some critics to call him the best actor of all time.

His later roles weren't all explosive. Think of his quiet intensity as a longshoreman in *On the Waterfront*, or as a mafia don in *The Godfather*. He couldn't play a role without seizing it. Inhabiting it. And finding the inner objectives for every act. (Well, almost every act—Hollywood being what it is, Brando also became Superman's father....)

Do men hide from their feelings? Some don't, but many do. No, your woman doesn't want a Stanley Kowalski ranting in her living room. But most women want their dates or partners to be open with their feelings, and are naturally drawn to a guy that is. Classically, that's what they need to get their own sexuality involved. An emotionally expressive guy has a leg up in the sex appeal category. Even the loner has to get into that scene sooner or later.

Be Smart and Funny

Actors get put in sticky situations. How they handle themselves makes the movie. Not surprisingly, most stars do well and prevail. They may use their bodies well, but it's their minds that get them their prizes, including, of course, the company of a woman. In the study mentioned earlier, women placed most value on intelligence and a sense of humor. When you think of actors and films you like, there probably aren't too many in which sharp thinking isn't a part of the formula. And in all but the most tragic stories, smiles are valued highly. Everyone likes to laugh, women included. That's why intelligence and a sense of humor are so high on the sex appeal scale.

Make her laugh. Impress her with your mind. The physical part will follow naturally.

Be Yourself

This is where our cinematic survey ends. The point is not to find mannerisms or accents to adopt. The real value of the movies begins when the movie ends. We walk out into the night and back into our lives.

Movies are just the latest form of the age-old tradition of storytelling. We watch and listen and learn.

Most actors possess all the traits mentioned above and so do you. Maybe some need developing; fortunately your life presents the opportunities for doing so.

Start with who you are now. Appreciate your strengths. Your shortcomings are probably not as important to others as you yourself envision them. Thinning hair? Not as tall as you'd like to be? Not as important to women as you may think.

Above all, learn how to be yourself. Be authentic. Go out and try for what you want. Build on successes and learn from failures. Be a man. That's what a woman responds to most.

SEX RESEARCH

The year was 1948. A group of scientists at the University of Indiana published surprising findings about human sexuality. The head of their team had realized that he could find more research about the sexual patterns of animals than about those of humans.

The man was Alfred Kinsey, and the study he organized shocked a nation. In one stroke, sex research came of age. Because his conclusions presented a different picture of American sex than was commonly assumed, critics attacked his work. Almost three quarters of older male teenagers having pre-marital intercourse? These were not the beliefs commonly shared over backyard fences in America. Remember, this was *before* the so-called Sexual Revolution!

At another extreme, and in our own decade, another sex study presented new conclusions. If the Kinsey study was revolutionary, the *Sex In America* study was counter-revolutionary. Now, it concluded, Americans are having less sex than popular notions propose (more on that study later in this chapter).

Between those two studies are others that have been welcomed by a curious public. When you read them and specifically about how they were conducted, you find different methods of research, ranging from informal magazine polls to rigorous methodology of high social science. Arguments for the accuracy and/or relevance can be made for all. And conclusions are debated endlessly.

Sex is too powerful an influence in our lives to leave in the dark. Ultimately, everyone has to make up his or her own mind about the impact of the findings of sex research. But curiosity is a strong human trait, especially in so strong an area as sex. So read on, and discover who's been doing what, how often, and why. It may not change your sexual behavior or opinions a bit, but then again, it very well might.

Our *Fit For Sex* survey of sex surveys concentrates on four classics in the field, starting with the most controversial sexual study of all time, the Kinsey research.

KINSEY (PERSONAL INTERVIEW)

Optimism swept the land as America began its postwar expansion. The massive effort of World War II was history, the baby boom was underway, and an unprecedented uniformity of cultural values reigned. Then right in the middle of this great momentum of economic energy and moral virtue fell the findings of Alfred Kinsey and his team of researchers.

His was not America's first sex survey. In fact he took pains to detail 19 previous studies. But the Kinsey study went far beyond anything published before, based as it was on 12,000 interviews from a variety of states (and age, educational, and professional segments of their populations). He researched both sexes, and published two books from his findings, starting with *Sexual Behavior in the Human Male*.

He expected criticism and opened his book by describing his procedures in detail. For advice about who and how to interview, he consulted a number of specialists from the fields of anatomy, anthropology, psychology, and many others. And talk about variety! He interviewed clergymen and journalists, lawyers and psychiatrists, bootleggers and hitchhikers, Harvard graduates and Indiana State Penal Farm inmates.

For nine years, he and his staff asked each person interviewed up to 521 questions ranging from their height to their preferences of masturbation, intercourse, even sexual involvement with animals.

Many professionals, he reasoned, would benefit from his work, among them psychiatrists, sex therapists, and sex educators. And many lay people interviewed wanted to relate their own sexual experience in an effort to learn more about that of their peers. Maybe there were others, for instance, who had experienced erotic arousal from non-sexual situations like riding a Ferris wheel, sitting in church, listening to band music, or reciting before a class.[154]

Fifty Years Young

Kinsey revealed some sexual attitudes and practices that were cutting edge fifty years ago—and some which remain so today. One example: Male orgasm without ejaculation. Many men today still aren't familiar with the possibilities that offers, such as advanced ejaculatory control and multiple orgasms. Yet there it was for all to see—reported in 1948![153]

They're (Gasp!) Masturbating!

Kinsey's research sheds light on a variety of sexual experiences. For example, what is normal regarding the number of ejaculations per week? For the first time, men could see how their married or single counterparts compared, or how ages 16-20 compared with forty-year-olds. They could also get a sense of the extremes at either end, such as one healthy male who reported one ejaculation in 30 years, or the lawyer who reported 30 ejaculations every week for 30 years![155]

And then there's masturbation! Shocking but true—boys and men were doing it freely! In fact 88% of boys aged 16-20 were slapping the monkey (even if they had other names for it). For single men, 53% still masturbated at age 50.[156]

Statistics like those highlighted a controversial reality: younger men engaged in frequent sexual "outlets," from masturbation to pre-marital intercourse. With Victorian sexual attitudes still predominant, and sanctioned marital sex not applicable, millions of men were forced into psychological conflict in attempting to deny their sexual impulses and adhere to a sexual abstinence that discouraged even masturbation.

As an alternative, Kinsey offered an overview of pre-Victorian western and other cultures where sexual play was socially accepted. He questioned the wisdom of having male sexual conduct prescribed by mothers and other women who generally report less interest in and experience with sex than younger men.

New information has emerged that questions Kinsey's personal life. Old grudges still remain about the accuracy of the sexual patterns he described. But there's no question about the enormous influence of his groundbreaking study. Much has happened in the fifty-plus years since he published his research, but not much that his study didn't in some way already bring to light.

We should thank Kinsey and his team and the enormous effort they made to differentiate what men actually do sexually from the infinite variations of what they "should" do. It wasn't the last word in defining the parameters of men's sexuality, but it certainly helped.

MASTERS AND JOHNSON
(LABORATORY OBSERVATIONS)

Where Kinsey briefly mentioned the physiological changes that occur during sex, William Masters and Virginia Johnson made them the centerpiece of their tremendously influential work published in 1966.

Rather than interview thousands of Americans to construct patterns of behavior among various groups, Masters and Johnson took a few hundred into the laboratory to study their sexual response firsthand.

The keyword was response, as in their book of the same name: *Human Sexual Response*.[157] Their purpose was to set the record straight about what happens when men and women have sex, and why they do the things they do when stimulated.

They began their study by comparing the overall differences in the way men and women respond to sexual stimulation. Their four-stage portrayal of sexual stimulation in both genders paved the way for a fuller understanding of women's sexual needs that would have profound consequences for men.

As described in *Afterplay*, the four stages are excitement, plateau, orgasm, and resolution.[158] They then analyzed the bodily changes that transpire during each of those stages in both sexes, such as breathing rate, blood pressure, flushed skin, etc.

Their study is strong in physiological detail if short in romance. If you're looking for details on the elevation of testicles in the excitement phase, Masters and Johnson is the place to go. Does an average size penis get proportionately larger when hard than one that's larger when soft? Masters and Johnson is still your source (and their answer is yes).[159]

They include a section on the changes older men experience during sex, such as the two phases of ejaculation gradually losing distinction. And they list the factors contributing to an older man's typical tapering off of sexual desire, such as monotony in monogamy, focusing on work or drink, etc.

Masters and Johnson cast more light into the sexuality of Americans, moving farther along the trail blazed by Kinsey.

HITE (ESSAY QUESTIONNAIRE)

A decade later, Shere Hite compiled yet a different type of male sex survey: anonymous answers to a mailed questionnaire. A wide variety of questions were asked and 7,239 men responded in writing, as opposed to the personal interview technique used by Kinsey. Responses were then grouped by subject. Varieties of subjects explore how men think and feel about sex. Do men feel angry at women? What are the emotional reasons that men like or dislike intercourse? Where do men stand on the subject of women's orgasms? Hite supplies the answers directly from the horses' mouths, as it were.

Her book contains a table tabulating the results of her survey. So if you want to know whether men like having sex with a menstruating woman, you'll find a specific answer: 67% of her sample said yes.[160]

The bulk of the study is excerpts of written responses to her questionnaire. She preferred this format because she wasn't primarily interested in establishing what is and isn't "normal" sexual behavior. Rather, she presents a group of men answering a question each in his own way. The reader is left to create his or her own conclusions.

Are You Happy With Sex?

In the Hite study, a woman is in charge. Does this affect the whole enterprise? You bet. As she explains in her introduction, she was interested in exploring why male sexuality is the way it is—especially when many men express dissatisfaction with it. She dedicates her book to the hope that men will stop walling themselves off in a one-dimensional sexuality based on emotional remove and a continuing war between the sexes.

Do you disagree with her assessment? Are you happy with your sex life? Are other men? These are the kinds of questions she posed, and the answers from a wide range of educational, geographic, and income segments of the American male population make for illuminating reading.

In terms of lifelong sexual fitness, one of the most interesting aspects of Hite's survey is men talking about how their sexual enjoyment and focus change from their 30's, 40's, 50's and beyond. Men report enjoying sex more as time goes by. In many cases, desire for an emotional connection grows and becomes an integral part of sexuality, interest in and skills with communication improve, and sexual desire itself increases!

This is must-read material for anyone who believes a man's sex life declines after his early twenties!

SEX IN AMERICA (SOCIAL SCIENTISTS AT WORK)

In 1994, another group of scientists compiled a sex survey called the National Health and Social Life Survey, published in a book called *Sex in America*.[161] They boasted a truly accurate sex survey produced with scientific methods which made previous surveys like Kinsey and Hite useless.

They also state right at the start that sex is not magic. One wonders what future surveyors will say about that, or that this survey only included people aged 18 to 59.

Their research paints a portrait of America very different from the media's picture of a sexually superactive citizenry. Begun to investigate the AIDS crisis, their survey not surprisingly presents a more conservative view.

But despite the alarming statistics regarding AIDS, the study, originally designed for governmental support, was ultimately rejected and had to find funding from private foundations. The authors found a silver lining, however, and were able to extend their survey past the narrow boundaries of the spread of STD's.

Their results indicate, as befits the work of social scientists, that sex is a more socially-oriented act than many presume. They see sexual patterns set more by shared social beliefs and customs rather than inner drives. They say that their findings confirm this, from whom people meet and choose as sex partners to the sexual patterns in marriage.

One trend that seems to have increased since the age of Kinsey is premarital sex. The *Sex in America* survey shows that four of five young adults have had intercourse by the age of twenty.[162] But overall, the study finds that Americans are having less sex than generally supposed, and are also generally content with monogamous sex.[163] In the age of AIDS and other STD's, these findings are neither surprising nor unwelcome.

SEX THERAPY

Call him Rudy. He's tall, muscular, outgoing, a successful lawyer, and he has a sex problem.

Rudy's problem—and the anguish it brings him—are all too common. He can't be inside his lover for more than twenty seconds before ejaculating. Yet he refuses to seek help. So he moves from one relationship to another, enjoying the chase, but when his problem becomes clear, and sometimes before, he shuts down and backs out emotionally. Worse yet, he's been doing this for six years since his divorce—all the while bragging in his health club about his fabulous sex life. Ah, men!

Unfortunately, Rudy's dilemma is not unique. An estimated 40% of American men have a problem with either premature ejaculation or erectile dysfunction (impotence) at some point in their lives.[164] Yet too many will deny their problem exists, sometimes even to themselves, and will avoid taking steps which could resolve it.

TAKE ACTION

In an ideal world, a man would realize why he's having a sexual problem and take appropriate action to correct it. Or his sexual partner would be understanding and willing and able to help. It does happen.

Often in the real world, however, all a man sees is a tangle of frustration and misery. He's too embarrassed to talk about it with even his best friend. And far from being understanding and helpful, his partner reacts with anger or turns away to protect her own sexual self-image.

Say it ain't so!

Well, commonly it *is* so—but doesn't have to stay that way.

There are hundreds of professionals specifically trained to help men like Rudy, with strong records of success in all types of sexual problems. In many cases the treatment is relatively short, without the long-term treatment often associated with psychotherapeutic counseling.

Rudy could help himself by stopping his denial of his problem and by starting to learn about it. Books, videos, web sites—there is more helpful information available now than ever before. He should bite the bullet and ask his doctor for advice. The embarrassment he might feel doing that would be nothing in comparison with the emotional turmoil his PE causes him already. Discovering whether a sexual problem has a physical basis is important to know.

If those steps don't help, he should think seriously about picking up the phone and calling (319) 895-8407. He'll reach the American Association of Sex Educators, Counselors, and Therapists (AASECT), where he can get the name of a qualified sex therapist in his location. If you ever find yourself struggling with a sexual problem you just can't move past, you should consider doing the same.

THINK LESS AND FEEL MORE

The field of sex therapy is surprisingly new, having grown largely from the work of William Masters and Virginia Johnson, whose efforts in sex research were noted earlier. As sex therapists, in the 1960's and 70's they promoted the sensate focus exercises on which most therapists still base their work today[165]—highly structured exercises beginning with non-sexual, nondemanding touch, the goal of which was to take pressure to perform out of a couple's sex life. They also introduced the squeeze technique, popular for slowing premature ejaculation.

In addition to that breakthrough work, more sex therapists have been refining other techniques in the field, adding individual psychotherapy, couples therapy, medication, hormone therapy, and more.

Sex therapist Eva Margolies, author of *Undressing the American Male*, notes that the answer to most male sexual problems is to "think less and feel more."[166] Others find the answer in building communication, or deepening intimacy in a relationship through both partners strengthening their own individuality.

SEX THERAPY IN THE FLOW

In previous chapters we examined specific sexual disorders: low desire, problems with intimacy, erectile dysfunction (ED), and premature ejaculation (PE). We'll review them briefly here, and see how they fit into the overall flow of sex, and sex therapy.

For men, an ideal sexual encounter flows from one stage to the next: desire, arousal, erection, penetration, orgasm, and resolution. There is no absolute connection between each of those stages and specific sexual problems. Yet there is a correlation between desire and arousal, erectile dysfunction and penetration, premature ejaculation and orgasm, and intimacy and every stage of sex.

Low Desire

Men and women confront many factors that can zap their sexual energy today: stress, depression, medications, poor overall health, and others. Whatever the cause, the outcome is the same: sexual desire at low ebb. Low desire might also relate to conflicts in a relationship or long-standing individual problems. It can occur on its own or in combination with premature ejaculation or erectile dysfunction. Its opposite—excessive sex drive—can also unsettle a man's life and sexual relationships and lead to sexual addiction. Either way, desire problems can slowly drain the life out of a sexual relationship, until ultimately threatening the well-being of an individual or a couple.

Only in the last twenty years has sexual desire been a focus separate from other sexual disorders. Helen Singer Kaplan, one of the sex therapists who originally identified it, states that up to 30% of people inquiring about sex therapy today do so for problems regarding low sexual desire or motivation.[167] She noticed that sex therapy based on sensate focus exercises weren't working when applied to low desire problems, and in some cases could even make them worse. In fact, some sex therapists today consider sensate focus exercises more useful as a tool for exploring a couple's problem, rather than treating it.

When a man's low desire predates his current relationship, the problem could point to long-standing conflicts about sex, women, or intimacy (which can also cause sexual aversion, or feeling disgust with and avoiding various aspects of sexuality). When the problem of low desire arises within a relationship, it's more likely to relate to his current partner.[168]

Of all the sexual problems discussed in this chapter, low desire can be one of the most difficult to change. In treating it, sex therapists employ many techniques, depending on the individuals and their sexual history. Individual and joint sessions, sex education, refining communication, specific sexual assignments, building intimacy, keeping sexual diaries, and recommending medications are all options considered helpful to move from low sexual interest to genuine desire, arousal, and satisfying sex.

Premature Ejaculation (PE)

Although a common and frustrating male sexual complaint, premature ejaculation is generally one of the less complex disorders. Here the "think less, feel more" approach may come to the forefront.

As discussed in the *Ejaculation* chapter, a typical PE problem is moving from arousal to ejaculation without much mental or physical awareness in between. Many early patients of Masters and Johnson enjoyed success through sensate focus exercises, coupled with specific approaches like stop-start and squeeze techniques. In recent years, some sex therapists have reported the successful combination of sex therapy and pharmaceutical drugs, using antidepressants such as Prozac and Anafranil, although potential side effects are always a concern.

Some sexual experts theorize that PE can result from early experiences, like intercourse or masturbation in which quick, penis-centered stimulation prevailed.

Sex therapist Eva Margolies notes two common causes of PE. First is "excessive sexualization," inappropriately intense reactions to sexual situations or possibilities.[169] She emphasizes the male tendency to intellectualize at the expense of bodily and emotional responses—investing casual touches with sexual undertones, and touching sexually in a hurried or uncaring way. Second is performance anxiety—a fear of failure and being judged negatively.

When there are no deep psychological issues calling for psychological counseling, or no apparent need for medication, sex therapists treat PE with exercises designed to help a man focus on feelings in his body rather on his mental expectations, needs, or fantasies. The goal, of course, is to slow him down—to slow ejaculation by slowing the whole flow from desire onward. The exercises are done at home, and are combined with office sessions and conversations about progress or frustration. The therapist can offer helpful feedback and other exercises to keep the treatment on the right track. When a man is in a relationship, sex therapists commonly prefer to see both partners together, except for periods when individual counseling is appropriate.

Even before specific sexual exercises begin, a therapist might recommend breathing or meditation to encourage the focus on physical sensations occurring moment to moment. Exercises like yoga or Tai Chi can also be helpful for grounding a man in his body and in the present.

Then a variety of exercises begin, often with a man simply touching himself in a non-sexual way, then arousing himself but stopping well before orgasm, which is often easier outside of partnered sex. Gradually, he learns to refine his ability to experience the whole range of sexual feelings when joined by his partner in non-demanding exercises leading to non-pressured arousal, erection, and penetration.

If these exercises fail to help him, a sex therapist can try alternative techniques personalized to the man and his needs, from medications to psychological counseling.

Erectile Dysfunction (ED)

While Viagra has helped millions of men suffering from erectile dysfunction, it doesn't work for everyone, is too expensive for many, and may mask underlying physical or emotional causes of the problem.

As with treatment for other male problems, sex therapy for erectile dysfunction starts with learning a man's sexual history. When physical problems such as cardiovascular disease have been ruled out, therapy often begins with exercises similar to those detailed for PE. Again, performance anxiety can be a significant obstacle. Non-sexual touching forms the foundation for subsequent exercises which progressively lead to successful and satisfying intercourse. Medications can help defuse tension, and as needed, individual and couples therapy is woven into sex counseling to overcome obstacles such as deep-seated negative emotions and reactions, and to integrate lessons learned into life beyond therapy.

Keeping Intimacy Alive

Sooner or later, sex without intimacy will become just going through the motions. A deep, emotional connection between lovers gives sex its enormous power to satisfy and heal and help keep an individual and relationship vital. When intimacy wanes, so can the strength of a relationship. A sex therapist can help partners find new ways to reveal important feelings and preferences in touch and sex, offer new techniques to spice up their love life, and encourage tenderness, and confidence in their ability to solve relationship problems as they arise. Intimate sex is an acquired skill, and a good sex therapist can help sexual partners learn it.

HANDS-ON SEX THERAPY

While some men might fantasize about erotic adventures with a curvaceous sex therapist, a certified professional would never be part of acting them out—but he or she might recommend someone who would, a decision never taken lightly, and never simply for a thrill.

The therapist might decide that a single man could learn valuable lessons from actually having sex with a woman trained to bolster his progress—a sex surrogate.

She wouldn't be an inexpensive option; nonetheless a sex surrogate can help various problems, such as sexual inexperience, physical handicaps, or the genital-centered disorders discussed above. Far from a one-night stand in a seedy motel, working with a sex surrogate usually involves a series of meetings in which the client learns, or relearns, how to expand sex beyond penis-centered stimulation. This is accomplished by working with relaxation exercises, communication, and simply tuning into the pleasures of sex rather than concentrating on performance.

ARE YOU READY?

Trying sex therapy is never an easy choice for a man. And it's one he shouldn't consider unless truly motivated, ready for change, and willing to work towards it. Mountains of male denial can't be crossed by sex therapy. And as noted above, some sexual dysfunction is too deeply rooted in psychological problems for change to be possible. In such cases, psychological counseling is needed for sex therapy to work its wonders.

Also, a man in a relationship needs to know whether his partner is willing and able to help, or too deeply part of the problem. It takes a strong woman to be able to look objectively at a man's sexual problem and see her involvement. Anger, resentment, or flight (emotional or physical) are common responses, preserving as they do her self-esteem, sexual or otherwise, in the face of sex gone sour.

A caring attitude will always arise when the relationship is essentially strong. She can find the motivation to work through her own psychological problems while he's working through his. Sex therapy can help reveal something beyond the passionate infatuation of pop songs or the embittered rut of relationship blues. Even deeply troubled sex can be transformed by the powerful beauty of making love.

SEX TOYS

Lovers occasionally get lost in grand expectations, try too hard to create passion, or otherwise lose sight of one simple reality: *sex is fun!* Responsible, consensual sex can be a blast! For many people, sex toys add a touch of spice to sex play.

But before going there, let's get serious and stay scientific. The generally conservative 1994 *National Health and Social Life Survey* of American sexuality included this surprising finding: over 20% of the men surveyed found using vibrators or dildos somewhat or very appealing![170]

Over one in five! Millions of American men! We can conclude that the subject of sex toys, although little discussed, is much more popular than generally believed. Of course that leaves many more millions not interested. They would no doubt express their lack of interest in anything other than natural endowments, and many men would be threatened by the idea of his partner using something that would make him "unnecessary."

If both partners are happy without toys, fine. But also fine is the desire to jazz things up with any of several erotic novelties. Whether you're interested in discovering sex toys for your own use or to boost your partner's pleasure, there's a growing world of possibilities to choose from.

We've looked at the power of intimacy, communication, and massage in deepening a sexual relationship. Now it's time to enlist all three while trying sex toys.

What is a sex toy anyway? Vibrators and dildos are the most popular, but the list includes body paints, cock rings, lubes, feathers, love bonds, and other objects all designed to maximize erotic sensations. Which of them should the beginning enthusiast try? Are they safe to use? Where can one buy them if not interested in braving the local sex shop? Good questions. Let's get straight to the answers.

ENJOY THE VIBES

Vibrators are the most popular sex toy. When the Lawrence Research Group published results of a survey of sex toy use, vibrators came out on top: 43% of sex toy users favored vibrators—followed by 30% for dildos, 19% for restraint devices, and 14.6% for penis stimulators.[171]

Dildos, or objects other than a real penis used for vaginal or anal penetration, claim the distinction as the oldest sex toy. Some vibrators are dildo-shaped, but a dildo doesn't vibrate.

Good ol' American ingenuity was responsible for the feel-good appliance called the vibrator. Cathy Winks and Anne Semans, authors of *The New Good Vibrations Guide to Sex*, cite 1869 as the year in which an American doctor introduced a steam-powered vibrator.[172] They further note that the vibrator was championed as a cure for "hysteria," the female complaint thought to arise from unreleased sexual tension. It's a bit difficult to picture the scene in a turn-of-the-century doctor's office with the country physician helping his patient to have a curing orgasm. Suffice it to say that patient-physician intimacy has been drastically reduced in the intervening years.

Since then, vibrators have been promoted as all-over muscle relaxers (and are still sold mainly as massage aids), leaving their sexual use a well-known secret. Only in the last twenty-five years have many sex therapists advocated their use, to heighten stimulation and help women learn to become orgasmic.

Though vibrators are used more by women, men also employ them to enhance sexual pleasure for themselves and their lovers. Although they enhance masturbation for both sexes, vibrators can add welcome energy to a sexual relationship stuck in a rut.

VIBRATING VARIATIONS

Many people erroneously equate a vibrator with the classic penis-like dildo. But vibrators come in a variety of shapes and sizes, and many are decidedly non-penile. There are two main types used for external stimulation: wand and coil, as well as attachments for each, and more specialized models for men. Power comes from either standard house electricity or batteries. Electric models tend to cost more, and avoid the hassle of replacing batteries. But the latter are more portable; even though most vibrators are used in the bedroom, the lack of a power cord can simplify things logistically.

Wand Vibrators

The best brands are sold in drugstores or electric appliance sources like department stores. Most are about 12 inches long, cylindrical, have an end resembling a tennis ball, and have two or more speeds.

Coil Vibrators

Picture a small electric cake mixer without the plate, bowls, or beaters; add vibrator attachments and you have a coil vibrator. They are heavier but quieter than wand vibrators. The vibrations are generally more intense and localized than those of a wand.

Attachments

Many types of attachments are available for each type of vibrator. A curved G-spot option directs the action to the sensitive front wall of her vagina. A two-pronged variation stimulates a clitoris and a vagina simultaneously. Other smaller attachments focus the vibrations on her clitoris. For specific penis stimulation, an expandable cup specifically fits over the glans of a penis.

Battery-Powered Vibrators

Lower-priced, gentler, and sometimes used internally, battery-powered versions are what most people think of as a vibrator. Many are designed to resemble and feel like a penis. Others are harder or rigid, smooth or textured, with many colors to choose from. Still others aren't penis-like at all, but rather small, egg-shaped vibrators connected to a battery pack.

For men only, a sleeve model allows a penis to be surrounded by pleasant vibes. There's a vibrating version of a cock ring, which is a ring worn at the base of the penis and historically used to maintain an erection by discouraging blood flow out of the penis. It is generally advised to wear one for only 20 or 30 minutes at a time so blood can recirculate.

CHOOSING A VIBRATOR

Needless to say, the best way to find the perfect vibrator is to try one. Or two. Whichever type you try, you'll soon get a feel, or feedback, for which area of genital stimulation works best. Then you can focus on the features (size, vibration intensity, durability, ease of portability, etc.) right for you and/or your lover. Enjoy, and don't worry about your lover choosing the vibrator over you. If she does, you'll know the relationship wasn't headed anywhere special anyway. Remember, the whole point of a vibrator isn't to focus on hardware, but rather enhance the fun!

FIVE TIPS FOR USING A VIBRATOR

Easy Does It

Including a vibrator doesn't change the progression of sex. Remember, women like to start slow. So why not begin by using a vibrator in its official capacity—as a massager. Try a back massage, foot massage, or whatever the moment calls for. Then approach and slowly focus on her clitoris, where many women go when using a vibrator themselves. Find out whether she likes direct or indirect clitoral stimulation. If you're using a variable speed model, start slow and turn up the vibes as the action heats up.

Keep It Clean

Clean a vibrator with soap and water (don't immerse in water). Air dry. Never go from anus to vagina without washing it. Using and removing a condom can make that transition easier.

Lubricate

Again, use vibe-free sex as a guide. Many sensations are naturally enhanced by massage oils. Use water-based lubricants for internal and condom-covered vibrators. Try a scented lube.

Experiment

Try different vibrators for different sensations. Soften the effect by wrapping the vibrator in a towel. Change positions. Ask your lover what she wants and listen to her answer.

Don't Overdo It

Margo Anand, author of *The Art of Sexual Ecstasy*, advises against overstimulating genital nerve endings with vibrators.[173] Others disagree. Let common sense be your guide.

THE OLDEST SEX TOY OF ALL

Since you've already got a penis, why would you want a dildo? While it's true that dildos are mostly a woman's toy, there are good reasons for a man to consider using one. If he's unable to have an erection, temporarily or otherwise, a dildo can stand in admirably (and can be strapped on if desired). If he ejaculates before she's climaxed, he might be considerate and help with the aid of a dildo. Or both partners might want totally safe penetration, either anal or vaginal, or possibly both simultaneously, in which case the right dildo is the perfect tool. And finally, a man can present his partner with a dildo for when he's away or busy—or just to prove what big-hearted, broad-minded stuff he's made of.

As with vibrators, there are many options from which to choose. Materials range from hard plastic to latex to soft rubber to silicone. Some are carved or otherwise textured. And of course hundreds of colors, sizes (width and length), and shapes are available. Some are easier to clean than others. Using a condom over a dildo insures safety from unwanted infections.

Also, as with vibrators, lubrication enhances the dildo experience. And here too, starting off slow and gentle is the best policy. Respect your partner's anatomy. Play safe!

SLIP AND SLIDE

There are a few good reasons to consider adding sexual lube to your bag of tricks. A woman's natural vaginal lubrication can decrease after menopause or due to other hormone-related factors like stress. Whatever the reason, having some sweet-smelling (or tasting) lubricant handy can keep the sexual energy flowing. It also helps whenever you use a penetrating sex toy.

Remember to use a water-based lubricant if you're using a condom or other latex barrier for safety reasons. With oils or oil-based lubricants you risk breaking down the latex and leaving holes for viruses or bacteria to get through. Water-based lubes are also less liable to stain sheets or clothing. Various brands are available which vary in consistency, from a thick gel to liquids. Look for lubes with nonoxynol-9 if safe sex is a concern. But be aware that it irritates some people's skin. Look for more information at your local sex shop or at one of the sources listed below.

RESTRAINTS AND MORE

Some sexual partners enhance their excitement by acting out fantasies, and bondage is one of the most popular. While commercial products aren't necessary here, leather restraints or padded versions add their own attractions for some enthusiasts. You can also just grab some rope or a scarf. The props are less important than the excitement generated within.

Ultimately, any sex toy is only as exciting as the sex in which it's used. The right attitudes and intimacy are the best starting point. Beyond that, anything that enhances the mood can work wonders. Videos, books, scented bath salts, massage oil, body paints, incense, and the classics mentioned above can all enhance the sensations, but can't create good sex in themselves. Good sex and fun sex toys go together best when communication is good and trust is strong.

SOURCES

If your local sex boutique doesn't have the sex toys you want (or it isn't a place you care to visit), mail order is the perfect alternative. The sources below are just a few of the many you can reach by mail, phone, or online.

Good Vibrations—938 Howard Street, San Francisco CA 94103
(800) 289-8423, or online at www.goodvibes.com

Blowfish—2261 Market Street #284, San Francisco CA 94114
(800) 325-2569, or online at www.blowfish.com

Adam and Eve—PO Box 800, Carrboro NC 27510
(800) 274-0333, or online at www.aeonline.com

Xandria Collection—165 Valley Drive, Brisbane CA 94005
(800) 242-2823, or online at www.xandria.com

SEXUAL MYTHS

Sex should always be great.

A woman should know what a man wants in bed.

Real men don't need intimacy.

The list goes on and on—grand illusions leading straight to frustration. Arguments. Low self-esteem. Even relationship dead-ends.

The good news is that most of these bogus sexual myths are losing their steam. After all, the weight and influence they carry stem only from repetition—and fear.

Real men! Who are they anyway? Aren't you a real man? Isn't every one of your male friends real too? Of course! We're all real men! And our sexual experience is real too. In fact, the only thing that isn't real here is the idea that an ideal man exists.

Sure there are times when we wish all sex was great. When we'd just as soon *not* get involved with the demands of intimacy, and when she damn well *should* know what we want.

But wish lists are different from reality. Facts are different from myths. Separating them is the job of...well...a real man like yourself.

Every myth has a germ of truth in it, and sexual myths are no exception. Hopefully by exploring the great sexual myths of our time, we can escape their negative influence.

Here then are seven of today's popular sexual myths with important truths waiting to be released, by you, in your personal odyssey through life.

SEVEN SEXUAL MYTHS

"Sex Should Always Be Good"

It certainly seems to be in movies and romance novels. Lovers tumble into bed, kiss like there's no tomorrow, moan and...well, you know the scene. But what about that complicated bra clip which breaks the timid guy's momentum and makes him feel like a jerk and sinks his confidence and so on? Or the numbing schedule the normally horny fellow's been hit with at work? Or her switching your sexual locomotive off the express rails onto a side track of talk? What then?

Then you're back in the real world, where sex has ups and downs just like everything else. The wise man accepts that, while the fool gets wrapped around the axle of how it *should* have been. Well, sit down a spell and consider the following truths that when accepted can contribute mightily to peace of mind:

- *Sex will stink from time to time.* That's not as hopeless as it sounds. In fact, terrible sex is a valuable message. Listen to what it says about you, your relationship, or (only after the preceding) her. Maybe it's time to spice things up a bit. Try a new position. Tell her you care. Or otherwise talk about what's going on. Remember, sex is an expression of your relationship, which has a life of its own and needs attention to thrive.

- *Don't make it a performance.* Basic advice to be sure, but it can't be overstressed. In fact, ask yourself whether the sex was lousy because you were trying to perform instead of staying connected emotionally with your partner. You'll know which is which, and which is better.

- *Sometimes just say no.* Some times are simply the wrong time for sex. Tell her so in language that stresses what *you're* feeling in non-accusatory language. Many a sexual problem starts with defensive pride driving sex instead of real arousal. Give yourself a break. Say no if that's what you feel. Who knows, maybe if you talk about it you might end up feeling a strong "yes."

"Real Men Don't Mix Sex and Intimacy."

Great advice in the sexual ballpark of forty years ago. Today, however, women expect more, and so should men. But too many still sneer at intimacy and the effort it demands. Less boisterously expressed, however, is that deep down they're afraid of intimacy.

Most men eventually discover that sex is much more than a hard dick, a fancy position, and a five-second orgasm. Sure, all that's nice, to say the least, but human sex is unique because it can lead men and women to new levels of satisfaction, personal growth, and ecstasy.

When we face our lovers during sex, we're connected in a way that's unique among our relatives in the animal kingdom. Maybe that's why a rear entry position can be such a turn on for both partners. It relieves us of everything that's difficult in face-to-face intimacy. It gets us closer to our roots in the animal world. Closer to raw sensation and pure genital release.

This is terrific. But being face-to-face brings us closer to something new in the evolution of sex: involving your whole self—attitudes and emotions as well as your body.[174] When you help to create the kind of shared sex based on all of who you are and can ultimately be, instead of what feels safe enough not to lose your erection, you've made a giant leap forward.

Sure, sexual skills can and must be learned. But not hidden behind! Intimacy presents the opportunity for learning how to be yourself, and more—for discovering yourself!

The satisfaction of connecting from a broader self is what beckons today. Since it's relatively new, it can feel somewhat uncomfortable. Once you've tasted the possibilities of intimacy though, you know there's no turning back.

"Real women know what real men want."

She should have a great body flooded with passion—and be a mind-reader too! Yes, and maybe tonight a magic carpet will carry you to the castle of the beautiful princess. Anyway, forget the mind-reading part—you'd be forever embarrassed if she knew the thoughts and pictures circulating in there! But admit it, you would like her to know exactly what you want sexually. Then you wouldn't have to face the discomfort of telling her—or worse yet, showing her.

Come on, be a man. Suggest some hot mutual masturbation. Of course first you'll have to know what feels good to you, well enough to show her. So you may have to spend some time researching that by yourself.

Okay, now it's time to tell her. It's the communication thing again. Because no, real men don't communicate mostly with their hips. They talk when necessary. And listen too. Because they respect the delicate bridges connecting them to others.

Again, enjoy the process. Getting to know her, and helping her to know you, is an ongoing journey, and a sweet one if you make the effort and take the time to taste it.

"Real Men Are Sexual Experts By Age 20."

Oh yes, we're such experts about life in general at age 20, right? So it follows that we're sexual experts too. Hah! The five-orgasms-a-night life might mean tons of sex, and some great learning experiences too, and a touch of smarts. But wisdom? Maturity? These take time. So does sexual maturity.

Learning to weave a woman's desires and yours is not easy. But every step along the way feels great when you're both committed to it. The challenge is remaining open enough to keep the discoveries coming. Being willing to try something new. Not standing on past accomplishments.

Ask a woman if she wants a technically skilled lover or an intimate partner. Unless she's just out for fun, most will pick the latter. Why? Because she's interested in you more than your genitals.

Forget the myth that we don't have to keep learning because we're all liberated now and everything's cool sexually. That's like suggesting you don't have to learn how to play a sport because everyone is just out there enjoying themselves. Balderdash! Keep learning. Keep listening. Keep great sex alive as you move through the many stages of relationship and life and love.

"Real men want sex twice today and twice tomorrow too."

Come on, be honest. After the post-graduation sexual lollapaloozas—or initial relationship fireworks—wear off and the years wear on, who could realistically pull off that sheer volume of sex ? For that matter, who would actually *want* that much sex? Let's keep a perspective here.

Take a guess: how many men in America are actually having sex four times a week or more?

8%! According to the 1994 *Sex in America* survey, that's the skimpy reality beneath all those hot stories you hear when men get together and impress each other with tales of erotic derring-do.[175]

The same survey showed 37% of the men responding have sex "a few times a month." Not far behind is the combined group of "not at all" and "a few times a year"—30%.

So statistically, at least according to one survey, most men are in fact not exactly sexual machines with throttle to the floor.

The good news is that even if we're having less sex than Hollywood's latest sexfest might suggest, American men enjoy the sex they do have.[176] Which is, of course, the bottom line. Whether we get all hot and bothered once a month or twenty, what really matters is—do we and our partners enjoy it? If you can answer that with a resounding "yes," you're in good shape, and so is your sex life.

But what about that nagging dream of sex day and night? Well, keep in mind that today's male porn stars are increasingly relying on Viagra to ensure that they can perform their celluloid wonders and keep the dream alive.

And the 7% of male 40-59 year-olds who *do* report having sex four times a week or more? Well, maybe it wouldn't hurt if they would stand up and tell the rest of us exactly what they eat for breakfast...just to satisfy our curiosity, of course.

"Real Men Get Hard Fast and Stay Hard Long."

Actually, human evolution has progressed far enough that the greatest male sexual secret can now be revealed: there's nothing wrong with your penis actually going soft during sex. True! Hopefully the revelation won't set off mass demonstrations and economy-jarring adjustments.

As we saw in *Midlife*, one of the surprises many men run into, and sometimes have trouble adjusting to, is the increased time needed for a full-scale erection at a certain point in life. There's a lesson here for men of all ages. Elapsed time from hitting the sheets to ramrod rigidity isn't a terribly important stat. Ask her! She often needs time to warm up to the whole idea of sex in general, let alone your accelerated vision of the act.

Okay, you're a super-stick-man. We get the picture. Nonetheless, there's wisdom in letting your penis decide when it's ready to rise. A soft penis is just as sensitive as an erect one. And being in her and feeling an erection unfold there feels most excellent!

Plus, even when you've arrived at advanced ejaculatory control or multiple orgasms (or if you're using a penis ring to sustain an erection), it's a good idea to let your erection relax a bit after 20 minutes and let the blood recirculate.[177]

The beauty of taking a little time to work into sex is that it allows you more time to get a feel for the situation at hand. Get a sense of where she's at. And let go of another sexual myth whose time has come and gone.

"Real Men Never Doubt Themselves Sexually."

Here we go again. Another high-flying sexual myth in search of an unsuspecting young buck (or an older one). The truth is that life has a way of throwing all of us curve balls. No matter how tall a man stands or how many notches in his bedpost, he can be rocked back on his heels from time to time. The assumption that we'll reach a point in life where we stand invincible to doubts and worries is a fine idea, but just an idea.

For example, consider our first experience of being too nervous, too tired, or too inebriated for an erection. Tough as the experience is, it's not unusual. How do we handle it? By allowing our self-esteem to crumble? Retreating into a deep inner cavern? Or putting it in perspective. Staying connected. Communicating.

We do have a choice, and in time maybe more of us will choose to explore what life presents us, instead of denying it, or putting up false fronts to defend against it. Confidence builds with success; sexual success is sustained in the long run by the beauty of intimacy.

SEXUALLY TRANSMITTED DISEASES

Once upon a time, ignorance was bliss. Then came the eighties and AIDS, and ignorance about sexually transmitted disease became catastrophic. Yet today, too few men realize their bodies are more easily infected by other sexually transmitted diseases (STD's) that are more common than AIDS. True, all can be treated, and most (but not all) can be cured. But with consequences ranging from the annoying to debilitating to deadly, it's no wonder many men would rather not think about these diseases.

Thinking is the vital first step toward preventing them. This chapter is intended to encourage that process. We'll look at the prevention, testing, and treatment of today's most common sexually transmitted diseases. Obviously, all of them directly affect your sexual fitness. Some men will need to put sex temporarily on hold. Others will end up wanting to swear it off altogether. But all men should step up and be responsible for their actions, and we'll detail how that is best accomplished.

STD's are transmitted in different ways. Some spread by contact with bodily fluid, others by direct contact with sores, warts, or ulcers. Because each of the diseases is different in risk and testing and treatment, we'll look at them separately. Taken together, however, they present challenges to all men today. Sometimes the challenge is simple, like remembering to have a condom ready, or learning how to happily integrate it into a sexual encounter. Sometimes the challenge is downright difficult, like telling your partner about your STD and accepting the consequences. But the bottom line is responsibility; being a man in the best sense of the word. Being smart and safe.

After that it gets easier. Then a man can immerse himself in the pleasure and passion!

STD'S TODAY

Before looking at the specific diseases, let's take a closer view of some of their implications.

In the early days of the Sexual Revolution, the main problems were syphilis and gonorrhea. Their consequences could be dire if left untreated, but all it took was a shot of penicillin and the swinging playboy was back in the game.

But today the chance of contracting some STD's can be as low as one in four incidents of unprotected sex.

With over 50 diseases classified as sexually transmitted, anyone

Symptoms To Watch for and Act On

Pain while urinating; sores, rashes, or warts on or near the penis; and fatigue or fever without known causes are all possible STD symptoms.

who is sexually active, or has partners who are sexually active, needs to know more about them. It might sound like a lot to learn, but the consequences are much more difficult, as anyone who has suffered one will tell you. We'll examine the most common, starting with the most notorious, the disease that made sexually transmitted diseases front page news.

AIDS

AIDS slowly weakens and destroys the body's ability to defend itself against a variety of other diseases. There is still no cure, although new treatments have reduced mortality rates.

Although it can be transmitted by infected needles and from mother to infant, sex is the virus's most common means of transmission. Unprotected anal or vaginal intercourse and oral sex can all pass the virus. When infected bodily fluids come into contact with cuts (and even microscopic tears in skin) transmission of the virus can occur. Blood and semen are the most common culprits, but no one has definitively ruled out urine, saliva, or sweat.

The World Health Organization estimates that 16,000 people worldwide are infected by the HIV virus *every day*. The number of Americans now HIV-positive is approaching one million (of an estimated thirty million around the world). And while the rate of incidence among homosexual men and intravenous drug users has fallen, AIDS among heterosexual Americans is rising. AIDS is more than a disease; it's an epidemic.

Optimism has been rising lately due to the effectiveness of the new antiretroviral drugs. While deaths from AIDS are decreasing, the rate of new infections has not fallen as dramatically.[178] Even in this country, where the treatment's cost is less of an issue than elsewhere in the world, problems remain with adverse reactions to the drugs and the virus developing drug-resistant strains. All in all, the best defense against AIDS now is what it's always been—safer sex.

AIDS progresses through stages. It may be months before tests reveal infection, during which time the disease can be transmitted. As many as nine years can pass before chronic symptoms appear, and eleven or more before late-stage immune system failure.

Many years of public education of the dangers of AIDS have boosted use of preventive measures, and caused a resurgence of condom use, but lately health officials have observed a surprising drift back toward apathy. Among younger users, ignorance and unrealistic feelings of invulnerability are still leading thousands of sexually active young adults to grief. Don't be misled by reports of recent medical progress. Take AIDS seriously, use a condom unless you know for a fact there's no risk, and enjoy life.

Tests: HIV RNA and HIV-antibody.

Treatment: Contact your doctor, a local health clinic, or call the AIDS hotline (800-342-2437), The Center for Disease Control (404) 639-3311, or the Sexually Transmitted Disease Hotline (800-227-8922).

One of the most dangerous aspects of STD symptoms is their absence. Some don't show up for months or years. That means if you're sexually active outside a tested monogamous relationship (meaning *both* partners have not had other sexual relations), you should consider being tested on a regular basis, possibly as part of an annual physical exam. If you suspect that you might have been exposed to an STD, or have questionable symptoms, see your doctor or visit a public health clinic *as soon as possible* for advice on when to test.

CHLAMYDIA

The most commonly reported STD, and especially prevalent among adolescents and younger adults, chlamydial infection can exist without symptoms. Yet it can cause prostate problems in men, infertility in both sexes, and pregnancy complications in women, who can pass the infection on to their children.

Chlamydia is caused by a parasitic bacteria called *chlamydia trachomatis.* It commonly infects the urinary tract. Male symptoms include a burning sensation while urinating or discharge from the penis.

But since those symptoms may or may not appear, the disease easily goes undetected. Sexually active men and women should therefore consider a yearly test for chlamydia, and when testing positive should notify their sexual partner(s) for their benefit and to avoid re-infection. Partners should undergo treatment simultaneously.

Tests: cell culture or blood test.

Treatment: antibiotics.

GENITAL HERPES

Genital herpes is a viral infection classified as type I or II. Type I is less common and generally causes sores around the mouth. Type II is more common and more dangerous, and is associated with sores on or near the penis. Pregnant women risk miscarriage and can pass the disease to infants, for whom it can cause death.

Outbreaks of blisters and sores can reoccur several times a year or remain dormant for months or years. Stress or other illnesses can initiate new outbreaks. This STD is most likely to be transmitted when sores are evident and the virus is shedding; however, transmission can occur without them. Only about half the people carrying the virus can feel symptoms of localized tingling or spreading pains which precede outbreaks. The initial outbreak is usually the worst. Symptoms include painful urination, penile discharge, and flu-like symptoms, including headache, fever, and muscle pains.

> **Safer Sexual Habits**
>
> A continuum of STD risk runs between abstinence (no risk) to unprotected anal and vaginal intercourse (high risk). Condoms, spermicides, dental dams, latex gloves, all reduce risk. Safer sexual activities range from phone sex, massage and mutual masturbation, to dry kissing (safer) to tongue kissing (less safe), to oral sex with barriers (safer) to without barriers (less safe), to the least safe sex, as mentioned above, anal or vaginal intercourse without condoms.

The sores or ulcers of genital herpes are sometimes confused with those of syphilis or chancroid. The Center for Disease Control and Prevention recommends testing for all three when one is suspected, and notes that all three have been linked with heightened risk of infection by the HIV virus.[179] A condom may not protect against transmission when open sores not covered are on the base of the penis.

Test: culture, scraping, blood test.

Treatment: An anti-viral medication called acyclovir can reduce symptoms and recurrence of outbreaks. Ointments can help reduce the pain.

CHANCROID

This is a bacterial infection with generally painful genital ulcers (sores) that can resemble those of syphilis and genital herpes. Its incidence in the United States has increased dramatically. Unlike genital herpes, chancroid can only be spread when sores are present.

Symptoms: sores appear up to 14 days after exposure. Flu-like symptoms and swollen lymph glands also possible.

Test: examination of sore scrapings, culture.

Treatment: antibiotics cure the infection and symptoms, and prevent transmission. Sores can leave scars despite successful treatment.

SYPHILIS

Syphilis is a centuries-old STD which still packs a potentially lethal punch.

The *T. pallidum* bacteria which causes syphilis spreads from the genitals through the body, producing stages of painless genital sores (which are sometimes hidden in men and women), then rashes, swollen glands, flu-like symptoms, and in later stages, blindness, organ deterioration, insanity, and death.

The earlier the treatment, the fewer complications are risked.

Test: blood test.

Treatment: antibiotics effectively treat the disease.

GONORRHEA

"The Clap" of yore, gonorrhea can strike with no symptoms or mild ones which include burning sensation on urinating or discharge from the penis. As you now know, these symptoms are shared by other STD's, which is why you need to see your doctor as soon as possible after noticing them. Recorded in ancient civilizations the world over, gonorrhea still infects over a million Americans each year. Untreated, the bacteria can produce prostatitis, arthritis, and meningitis.

Test: culture of penile discharge.

Treatment: antibiotics.

GENITAL WARTS

Look at a textbook photo of genital warts and you'll get serious about preventing STD's. The genital/anal region can be covered by warts which are about as far from eroticism as possible (although they're most commonly too small to see without magnification). Human papillomavirus (HPV), which can be present without external warts, has been linked to cancer of the penis in men and of the cervix in women.

Another centuries-old sexually transmitted disease, HPV is treatable but not always curable.

Test: visual examination

Treatment: warts are removed by solutions or gels (self-administered), or burning, freezing, laser or traditional surgery, injections, or combinations of the above. Treatment for warts on the penis is recommended to minimize the risk of future penile cancer.

HEPATITIS

Up to 60% of hepatitis B (HBV) is transmitted sexually, and the STD is now infecting almost a quarter of a million people annually in the United States. Symptoms include fatigue, flu-like symptoms, and gastrointestinal problems. Liver infection and death are the most serious threats. Anti-viral drugs are showing promise in treating non-acute cases, and a vaccination is available.

Hepatitis A (HBA) is less common, but it can also be transmitted sexually. International travel and/or contaminated water or food are among other causes of contamination. Liver disease is not linked to HBA, and again, besides safer sexual practices the best preventive action is a vaccination.

STRESS

A forty-something man meets his father for lunch. The son describes how stressful his marriage is, and how helpful counseling has been for helping sort through his feelings. His father, impatient and irritated, cuts him off in midsentence.

"Marriage is just another job," he blurts out, wagging a finger at his son. "Just take charge, bring home the bacon, and get out of the house as often as possible. For my generation, stress never existed."

While we might wonder about the nature of his marriage, apparently he has found a successful way to cope with stress, since he's quite old and apparently fit.

Stress is a physical reaction to a perceived threat. Something one man finds intensely threatening leaves another man untroubled. Sadly, this father's description of his generation is, though over-generalized, largely correct. Many of those fathers worked hard, drank hard, and didn't have the time or inclination to entertain ideas like stress. Unfortunately, many also died from the impact of unacknowledged stress.

Our lives are even more complicated than those of our fathers. Economic security is less assured. Many wives are working hard in their own stressful careers. In this high-speed, high-tension world, how can a man minimize or eliminate stress—including its impact on his sex life? And for starters, what exactly *is* stress?

COPE OR CRUMBLE

For century upon untold century, when the woolly mammoth attacked, a hunter was flooded with hormones that supercharged his mind and body. Our intrepid warrior stood firm with spear ready for action, or, when eye-popping discretion prevailed, sprinted in the opposite direction at full speed. Scientists call that the fight-or-flight response. But today? A guy's in bed with his wife or girlfriend and she demands sex again before he's ready (it happens more than men care to admit). Different situation, same response—threat perceived, stress chemicals released. Unfortunately, the penis first needs to be relaxed in order for blood floodgates to operate properly and cause an erection. No dice this time.

Without an effective attitude and coping technique, the poor fellow in question can mark another frustrating episode in the stress column. Sexual tension is one thing, and a welcome part of the process, but feeling threatened is something else altogether. It might be an erection problem now, and further down the road, lead to a reduced sexual desire problem too.

So stress interferes with sex directly. Also, long-term stress causes other physical complaints which can indirectly affect sexual desire, arousal, and performance.

It's even trickier today, murkier in a way, because many of our stresses tend to be generated within ourselves. After all, not too many men today commute to a job hunting woolly mammoth. Today, we're often victims of our own emotions, ideas, memories, and expectations,[181] which can cause the same reactions once reserved for external threats.

For health and sexual fitness, you need to be able to recognize stress reactions—and know how to neutralize them. Eventually, you should learn how to avoid them in the first place, but given today's world, that's not always possible.

> ### Stress-Related Disorders
>
> One stress expert estimates that up to 90% of all physical ailments and conditions are in some way related to stress.[180] Sexual dysfunction is certainly one. As you can imagine, sex is certainly affected by others: tension headache, back pain, jaw tension, chronic pain, migraine headache, anxiety, depression, high blood pressure, skin problems, allergies, asthma, arthritis, stomach pain, digestive disorders, diarrhea, frequent colds, infectious diseases, cancer, stroke, fatigue, and profuse perspiration, just to name a few.

RECOGNIZING STRESS

Boom! The boss just promoted someone else into a position you expected. Your father died. Your wife informed you she's moving out. Those are major league stress factors. But others contribute their share too: your wife announces she's pregnant, or a new term at school, or the first days of retirement. All potentially hard on your system. Your mind, emotions, and body are all affected.

Most immediately, your blood pressure, heart rate, blood sugar and muscle tension all jump, prepping you for action. But what most people

Guy Stress

Gail Sheehy, in her book *Understanding Men's Passages*, notes that men have more intense physical reactions to stress than women, and are more sensitive to emotion-based stress.[182] Once our inner alarms are tripped and the stress hormones spill into our bloodstream, our blood pressure spikes higher and stays there longer.

Add some classic male denial of upsetting emotions (especially anger or hostility) to a tendency to hold them in rather than share them, and you have a recipe for disaster: heart disease, depression, or erectile dysfunction.

think of as stress is not so much those reactions as when they repeat over time, often for reasons without simple solutions. That's chronic stress, and it's dangerous.

Consider, for instance, your heart. It can easily handle the increased demands of tension—unless it occurs repeatedly without an appropriate physical reaction of fight or flight. In the long haul, stress reactions take a toll: chronic high blood pressure, headaches, or higher cholesterol levels. The whole person is affected.

Mentally, stress can cause anxiety, memory, and concentration problems. Emotionally, it promotes feelings of tension, restlessness, fear, irritability or depression. Physically, look for teeth grinding, constipation or diarrhea, headaches, fatigue, nausea, reduced immune function, sore muscles (and inappropriately flexed muscles that can interfere with erections) and reduced sexual desire.

The next two questions follow naturally from there: how can a man defuse stress he already feels, and how can he avoid it in the first place?

NINE STRESS-BUSTING TECHNIQUES

As we've seen, stress factors abound. But whenever they muscle into your life, you *can* neutralize their impact and stay on track. Your stress-busting options range from quick-acting "emergency" techniques to longer-term stress avoidance. They're all beneficial and all encourage health and fitness in daily life—and nightly sex.

Move

Sometimes you'd just like to reach out and punch someone. But fighting is about as appropriate in the modern world as dragging a woman around by her hair. Try flight instead. Fortunately, it still works wonderfully well in relieving stress. Aerobic exercise, such as running, biking, roller blading, or swimming is a premier stress-buster. Regular workouts are the closest you'll find to physical immunization against stress. By strengthening and toning your cardiovascular and muscular systems, you make yourself more resilient to external stresses. But don't create a stress-generating regime. Sometimes a quick walk at work at lunch or break times can provide a great outlet for stress-born tension. Again, the exercise doesn't have to be exotic: mowing the lawn is a great way to shake off someone's bad attitude.

Breathe

One of the simplest yet most effective stress-reduction techniques reverses the tense, shallow breathing caused by stress. There are many types of breathing techniques, like simply counting breaths from one to ten, backwards from fifty to 0, yogic breathing through alternate nostrils, or full breathing from the bottom of the lungs upward. All can help slow your stress-heightened heart rate and other stress responses.

Meditate

Dr. Herbert Benson popularized meditation as stress relief in his breakthrough book *The Relaxation Response*.[183] His research proved the hypothesis that our body has, in addition to the tensing fight-or-flight response, an opposite, relaxation response, which has become overtaxed due to the sheer number of stresses built into modern life. His work bridged more than one wide gap: first, it brought into focus the health impact of the mind on the body, and it brought ancient religious techniques of meditation into the modern laboratory. The result: a proven technique to counter the effects of stress. High blood pressure was the main condition he sought to counter, with success.

His method, derived from age-old meditation techniques, was fourfold, and has been adopted and adapted by many:

- *Begin with quiet.* A quiet room, a quiet place outdoors, a quiet time of day minimize distractions.
- *Be comfortable.* Sitting is the preferred position, but you don't need the specific postures of oriental traditions. On a chair, kneeling, or sitting cross-legged all work. Keep your back straight.

- *Find a mental focus.* An object, a sound, a word, breathing, whatever feels natural for you. Dr. Benson substituted simple, familiar sounds for those of specific meditation traditions, and found them as effective.

- *Adopt a passive attitude.* Let thoughts come and go. Simply bring your attention back to whatever you're focusing on. There is no need or reason to judge yourself in this process. This is not a competition; in fact it balances the intensely competitive environment in which so many of us work and play.

Meditation is a perfect antidote to our rush-here-rush-there, do-this-do-that lifestyles. It's passive. It stops our constant flow of energy outward and allows our bodies and minds to stop and renew themselves with their innate, nourishing energies. Meditation is one of the most powerful and healthy tools you can use to foster short- and long-term health and fitness. Try one of the various meditation groups near you.

Stretch

In the fight-or-flight response, blood pressure rises, muscles tense in preparation for movement, and blood flow to the digestive organs is decreased. These are just some of the responses which can become chronic with constant stress. Stretching can help reverse them. Explore all the possibilities from simple stretches, like slowly circling your head or raising your shoulders, to the mother of all stretching systems—yoga—until you find those that work for you at work and at home. Headaches, neck aches, and backaches are often clear messages that you need to stretch to relief tension. Ignore them at your peril.

Medicate

With powerful anti-anxiety and anti-depressant drugs on the market, many people are finding stress relief from a pill. While they might be appropriate for some conditions and some people, pills don't address underlying conditions. Like all pharmaceutical drugs, they attack symptoms without supporting your body's healing systems. Some drugs hailed as breakthrough cures end up causing toxic side effects and adverse reactions. For example, Prozac is a popular antidepressant which can reduce both sexual desire and performance,[184] among other known side effects.

Natural alternatives like herbs can work too in reducing the impact of stress, but without side effects. Extracts of valerian, ginseng, licorice, and kava are four that the respected herbalist Kathy Keville recommends as a stress-busting brew.[185]

Connect

Visit your brother or sister, talk with a friend, or just pet a dog! Research shows that social networks provide crucial support against stress and its ill effects on health. From death rates to colds, people who live in isolation are much more likely to suffer.[186] Whether you're married with a large family or living alone, there are times when a trained therapist can help you spot attitudes and feelings that create rather than diffuse stress. Don't be too macho to benefit from his or her input.

Float Like a Cloud, Strike Like a Snake

Imagine a set of slow standing movements that combine meditation and exercise, promote health, and have been tested and refined for thousands of years. You've just imagined a real-world system called Tai Chi Ch'uan, or more commonly, simply Tai Chi.

Developed in China by Taoist masters, many of its postures were created by early practitioners closely observing the natural world, hence posture names including clouds, snakes, storks, and others. Tai Chi is easy and enjoyable to do, a potent and natural stress-buster, and becoming a common sight in many of America's parks. At advanced levels it has martial arts applications, but most people just enjoy its unique combination of calming and strengthening benefits. Most cities have groups and lessons available. Look in your phone book under Tai Chi or Martial Arts.

Think creatively

Don't settle into mental ruts that only perpetuate stress. Psychologist Suzanne Kobasa recognized three attitudes associated with successful stress management.[187]

- *Think of stressful situations as a challenge.* When one approaches difficult times with that attitude, they are no longer threatening. Your energy becomes positive, and a healthy, nonstressful response is more likely.

- *Make a commitment.* When you confront a challenging situation on behalf of others, your effort gains additional meaning. Working for the benefit of family, friends, or colleagues all help, adding to the possibility of successfully attaining a goal and avoiding stress.

- *Be in control.* A feeling of helplessness compounds stress. When you feel like you have the power to control a situation, you're aware of options that make your efforts more likely to succeed. Being in control of yourself is important too, because you can't control every situation you come upon.

Make Love

Lastly, there's the delightful alternative of combining all of the above—in bed! Sex is, among other things, a terrific stress-buster. In this context, a quickie can be just what the doctor ordered. But in order for this prescription to apply, your lover should be receptive to a wide range of sex scenarios, from lengthy passionate extravaganzas to the occasional quick roll in the hay. But be careful, if you overuse this card you might be reduced to solo sex, stress-reducing and otherwise.

TANTRIC SEX

Okay, time to shift gears...decelerate...stop the headlong rush from point A to point B...and consider true sexual gold. Forget foreplay and intercourse and afterplay as you know it. Unplug the clock and all it represents. Take a deep breath. Relax. There's only one time frame here—the present. And in it you'll discover a different kind of sex altogether. Consider revising your notion of a good orgasm, good connection with your lover, and sexual satisfaction. Consider revising them all upward.

Admittedly, this chapter won't be for everyone. That's okay because it's not meant to be. And don't be surprised if dissatisfaction with sex-as-you-know-it drives your curiosity about what this area of sexuality offers. If you've ever felt disappointed with sex, and wondered if there was more to it, then it's no mistake you're here. Because yes, there is more to sex than machine-like pumping, me-first demands, and post-coital emptiness. Much more! In retrospect you may find yourself smiling at having felt so negative about something you intuitively know to be so positive. In the long run, people end up thankful for some pretty disillusioning experiences they've had along the way. That's life!

Conversely, maybe you've had a taste of something special that you can't begin to explain: starting out in normal sex and ending up with ecstatic moments, expansiveness, oneness. Quite simply you'd like more of the same.

One reason for looking is not better than another. What matters is the looking—and, of course, finding.

GOING DEEPER

Before introducing tantric sex in particular, we might ask what spiritual sex in general would be. Well, we all know what sex is, and we all know what spiritual is. Or do we? What *does* spiritual mean anyway? Well, a ton of definitions exist, some loaded with vast histories of holy conflicts, inquisitions, and other bad news. Then there are the well-publicized stories of American gurus entangled in questionable sexual intrigues.

Maybe one usable definition of the spiritual is that which connects you with something larger than yourself, your desires, or your partner—a sense of union or oneness with everything.

Now rest easy, you won't find an attempt here to sway you with some new-fangled tangle of spiritual nonsense. After all, our subject is sex. Sexual fitness. How far you take it is purely up to you. But suffice it to say that you can travel a remarkably long way before reaching the far side of sexuality's potential.

SEX IS GOOD

Originally a movement that grew alongside the ancient spiritual traditions of India, tantra was primarily a path to spiritual enlightenment. What set tantric texts and masters apart, however, was their insistence that the body and its sexuality was not a distinct matter or separate consideration from the highest spiritual realizations. To the contrary, they argued, sexual energy is an integral part of everyone's physical, mental, emotional, and spiritual existence, and must be utilized in, and not set apart from, the quest for ultimate wisdom.

That distinct vision still exists in various tantra forms. Some have argued that tantric teachings in the West today have been diluted beyond recognition in tantric workshops and couples weekends. But we Americans are a practical group, always taking what we need from a wide variety of sources. So what harm results from a relationship benefiting from enhanced intimacy of tantric exercises? Or a man or woman deepening his or her sexuality and intimacy with this age-old wisdom? Not to worry, the further spiritual dimension will always be there, beckoning to those ready to respond and follow sex to its ultimate potential.

TANTRIC NUTS AND BOLTS

Tantra, like other Eastern traditions, presents a path to unity, a merging with the absolute. A practitioner first unifies him- or herself, merges with a partner, and finally experiences a sense of oneness with all of creation. Tantra's paths combine sex with ritual, meditation, exercise, controlled breathing, dance, and yoga.

As Margo Anand points out in *The Art of Sexual Ecstasy*, the path to sexual ecstasy doesn't begin with finding an ideal lover, it begins with accepting who you are right now.[188] That includes being able to accept your body and mind as they are in the present, and letting go of feelings of guilt and shame.

Since spiritual sex represents a different approach to sex, it can help to acknowledge that fact with a special atmosphere, if not a different room devoted to it. The use of candles, incense, soft music, and natural objects such as plants and rocks can help create the effect of a sacred space, in which a new approach to sex is practiced and appreciated.

Don't allow distractions to interfere with your delight. Find a time when you won't be interrupted. Unplug the phone.

To begin, we arrive again at the practice of meditation.

HIGHER SELF-PLEASURE

Meditation can help you settle down, relax, and be fully open to what sex has to offer. If you're new to it, meditating can be simple and informal. In fact, you might want to begin by just lying down. Otherwise, sit with a straight back and listen to whatever sounds or smells reach your ears, nose, and closed or lowered eyes. Be aware of your breathing. If you're lying on the floor, consciously give your full weight to it: allow it to support you.

When you're ready, follow your breathing. This is not a test or competition of any sort. Naturally your thoughts will wander: "What shall I cook for dinner, what did so-and-so mean by that, etc..." Simply bring your attention back to your breathing when you notice your attention has wandered. Follow your breathing in your nostrils and down into your chest and abdomen and back out through your nostrils. Your abdominal muscles move like steady and slow bellows when your breathing is relaxed and natural.

After ten to twenty minutes of that, silently acknowledge your love and acceptance for yourself. If you feel moved to do so, say a prayer of thanks to God, the Higher Power, Great Spirit, or whatever grounds your spirituality.

A basic tantric belief holds that the body and all its functions are aspects of the divine.[189] Yet as we saw in *Masturbation*, guilt is a common obstacle in exploring our own body and sexuality. Hopefully it will fade with other distractions as the journey continues. Everything so far plays an important part in laying a strong foundation for what follows.

BRING UP THE BLISS

Transforming genital pleasure into mental ecstasy is the heart of tantra. Imagine not merely having more powerful or longer lasting genital orgasms or more of them (although don't be surprised by them either); rather, look for sexual energy to be transformed in its move from the genitals to the heart and on to the mind. That specific energetic transformation takes in the chakras, "each of which is both a generator and a reservoir of energy and psychic consciousness."[190]

Starting from the first chakra at the base of the spine, the next highest is the second (genital area), third (behind the navel), fourth (heart), fifth (throat), sixth (between the eyebrows), and seventh (crown of head). The chakras are connected by channels of energy, like the energy paths called meridians in Chinese acupuncture. Each chakra is associated with one human function, such as the third, behind the navel, with the digestive system. So you can accept them as a literal system (which is difficult when judging from the western scientific point of view), or as a symbolic ladder in the human body from the "lower" centers to the "spiritual" seventh chakra, our link to the cosmos. Tantra is the path which activates this system with sexual energy, and therefore transforms it into spiritual oneness and bliss.

We can begin the move toward ecstasy by learning to move our sexual energy upward, beginning with self-stimulation. Massage oil will help. The point is to pleasure yourself and progress toward orgasm, but instead of ejaculating, stop and move the energy from your genitals to your entire body through what Anand calls the Inner Flute,[191] or sexual energy pathway. Through a combination of breathing and flexing your PC muscle, you move the sexual energy first up to your heart and then to your brain.

THE SKY'S THE LIMIT

When you have begun to feel the energy rising, you're ready to apply what you've learned to the intimacy of partnered sex. The preliminary steps are the same, starting with meeting in a space with sacred objects and atmosphere, quiet, and thankfulness. Begin by just being with each other, as in meditating together or giving each other a gentle massage. Again, what's important is to give yourselves time to relax and come into each other's presence as fully as possible. Open communication can help remove any reservations, expectations, or other obstacles.

One form of intimate communication is a shared meditation while lying front to back in the "spoon" position. Either partner can be in front. If your partner lies in front of you, gently hold whatever part of her feels good to both of you. There are two ways to utilize breathing.[192] In the first, you breathe in and out in unison, inhaling, gently holding the breath, exhaling, holding the breath, and repeating. Alternatively, when one partner breathes in, the other breathes out. Try both. More advanced, shared chakra visualization can create a spiritual bond as well as an expanded sense of presence and intimacy.

Then you can proceed to the same exercises outlined above in individual practice. Moving apart from the spoon position, one or both partners can pleasure themselves to the brink of orgasm, then stop and draw the energy out of their genitals and up their inner flute. Or one can pleasure the other and vice versa. In time you learn not to simply move to orgasm, but to spread the sexual energy up through the body.

When you're ready, you can make love in any of the positions outlined in *Intercourse*, still with the intent of deep intimacy and to withhold ejaculation and move energy up the inner flute. Finally, try the position often associated with tantric sex. She sits on your lap and you breathe and move in harmony, both tightening and loosening your PC muscles, rocking pelvises, and breathing the energy upward. When your genitals and mouths are connected, an energetic circuit can close, circulating through both of you, and the sky's the limit to ecstasy.

EIGHT TANTRIC TIPS FOR HIGHER SEX

Focus on presence and connection rather than maximizing performance or orgasm.

Develop intimacy with tender words, touch, dance, or whatever opens the channels of communication.

Exercise your PC muscles (see *Kegel* for instructions) and practice tantric breathing too (inhale while contracting PC muscles and bringing sexual energy upward along the inner flute).

Don't overdo it. Make sure you're fit and strong enough before trying advanced or prolonged tantric positions.

Practice makes perfect. Don't expect magic when just starting. Give yourself time to develop.

Learn to withhold your ejaculation—not every time you make love but enough to feel the difference it makes.

Find a teacher. Knowledge of tantric sex has traditionally been transmitted from teacher to student directly. Because of its popularity in the West today, finding a teacher is easier than ever. Be careful, however; just because teachers use the name "tantra" doesn't mean they're qualified to teach or to be trusted. Exercise caution. Ask for references.

Be thankful for the vast rewards of tantric sex.

TAOIST SEX

Taoist sex is China's contribution to the world of eroticism. While we can find old paintings that look suspiciously like China's contribution to early pornography, that's probably just our modern take; true Taoist sex is as much about health and longevity as pleasure. We Westerners are just getting used to the idea of sex and health as happily coexisting, after living for centuries with the idea that sex is dirty and best swept under the rug.

Along with its unique approach to sex, China also has a long history of using acupuncture, a remarkably non-invasive form of healing based on the body's life energy, *chi*, flowing through pathways called meridians. As noted in *Tantric Sex*, those meridians can be used to move sexual energy and pleasure from the genitals through the body. While Taoist and tantric sex share many features, there are differences, as we'll see shortly. Please be advised that both chapters are strong stuff. Consult your doctor or other qualified health professional before trying the exercises described.

GO WITH THE FLOW

As old as that phrase is, it still rankles many people because of its association with flower children, laziness, and amorality. But there's more to going with the flow than that. For one thing, there's Taoism, the ancient Chinese philosophy that grew from close observation of the natural world. The Tao (pronounced "dow") is the universe, nature, and also its flow and natural process.[193] Taoist sages uttered paradoxical nuggets describing how humans can best live according to natural law. And somewhere along the way, they developed specific ideas about sex, in part from tantric influences flowing eastward from India.[194] But again, the local foundation remained strong. A central pillar of Taoist sex has always been how it relates to health and longevity.

SAVE THE SEEDS

While health is a concern for men of all ages, relatively few invest a lot of thought in longevity, at least until middle age. And still fewer connect it to sex. Not so with the Taoists. Sex, health, and longevity are intimately bound, and to find out why, we arrive at something we've already noted: the separation of orgasm from ejaculation. But here we get a new twist. The bad news, from the Taoist point of view, is that indiscriminate ejaculations weaken a man and cause premature aging; the good news is that doesn't mean men can't enjoy spectacular sex, including multiple and whole-body orgasms. Details follow.

Mantak Chia, who has popularized Taoist sex in the west through books and a network of teaching centers, sums it up this way: "In all forms of life, the reproductive act exhausts essential energies."[195] In looking at everything from trees to salmon to insects, he sees the same lesson: sexual function plays a central role in all life forms, but when its work is done, physical decline is the next step. In humans, however, two important differences reign supreme regarding sexuality: first, sex all year (and not seasonally as with our relatives in the animal world), and secondly, we seem to be unique in having a spiritual side, which has unique implications for human sexuality.

Humans can make love a lot—all year long and every day if desired. Unfortunately, from the Taoist perspective, such sex will eventually weaken a man and age him prematurely. But humans also have the singular ability to have sex in such a way that supercharges pleasure *and* the body. Intense, spiritual sex strengthens the body, and the mind, and the spirit.

Taking the Yin with the Yang

The principle of polarity also lies at the heart of Taoist sex. The ancient sages saw that everything in nature has an opposite but complementary form: winter/summer, night/day, hot/cold, man/woman. And more, as the famous yin yang symbol demonstrates, everything contains a bit of its opposite. This is important for men. You do have a feminine side. Not only is that natural, and necessary, but only in accepting it and acting from it in part can you become whole. Yes, true intimacy and deep connection are challenges for some men, but therein lies the path to their ultimate wholeness and satisfaction. You can still be a regular guy and spit and flex your muscles and watch hockey on TV. But why not talk to a woman when she needs it, listen, and take the time to care about her feelings and yours too?

When you learn to accept the feminine as well as the masculine within yourself, you'll find yourself less impacted by the battle of the sexes in your outer life as well.

SUPER SEX FOR SUPER LONGEVITY

Western science tells us that male sex hormones are produced in the testicles. The Taoists would add that a vital life energy is produced there as well, and that life energy is either lost with ejaculated sperm or retained when sperm is retained. And more, Taoist sex teaches us that hormone production is linked with sperm retention or loss.

As we saw earlier in the book, certain male hormones begin to decline as a man approaches middle age. Some researchers thereby hypothesize the existence of a male menopause leading to a decline in muscle mass, hair loss, wrinkling skin, and other manifestations of aging.

Daniel Reid, author of *The Tao of Health, Sex, and Longevity*, writes that by using Taoist sexual practices vital energy and hormone production can be boosted and aging can be slowed.[196] In other words, sex can be a powerful anti-aging strategy.

SEX IN ORBIT

Back to the flow. Acupuncture heals because it frees the flow of bioelectric energy through the body, which circulates like electricity through home wiring. From the Taoist perspective, erotic energy can be circulated through an energy channel from right behind your testicles up the spine to the brain and down your face to the depression between your mouth and nose. Another channel extends from there down the front of your body to the same area, right behind your testicles, called the perineum. Together, those two channels create a circuit of bioelectric energy, which Chia calls the Microcosmic Orbit.[197]

When sexual energy runs through this circuit, it carries its life force with it, nourishing and strengthening your body. And not coincidentally, you feel its energy throughout your body instead of just in your genitals. From the Taoist perspective, health and longevity are enhanced when this concentrated life energy is circulated often.

So the Taoists present a choice. Either we can run this essential life energy through our bodies—or out our penises when ejaculating. Of course they advocate the former. And that means controlling ejaculation. Orgasms, thumbs up; frequent ejaculations, thumbs down.

Again, the trick is learning how to have an orgasm without ejaculating. And though there are similarities to tantric sex here, there is a uniquely

Taoist slant on the subject too. The place to start is a new, wholly pleasant, and simultaneous combination of self-pleasuring, breathing, exercise, massage, and meditation.

PREPARE FOR BLISS

Self-Pleasure

Okay. You've created a comfortable, uninterrupted space and time. You're taking the first step toward transforming sexual energy into healing whole-body energy. We're talking pleasure here. In this country, at this time, we have localized much of our sexual pleasure in our genitals, or more specifically, in our penis. That's understandable, since, hey, it feels pretty darn good. But the first step in expanding our sexual horizons is to start feeling the rest of our body. Start with simple touch. Lay your hand on your chest and feel its warmth, its movement with breathing. Now how about your belly, thighs, and something that might be new to you called the perineum? Read on.

Massage

After simply feeling that magnificent body of yours, try rubbing, preferably with massage oil, the same way you'd rub your lover. Maybe staying with this will be enough for now. If not, explore your penis, testicles and the erogenous area you may not have discovered before: the perineum, between your testicles and your anus. What's interesting about this area is that it's over your prostate and PC muscle. Orgasm is initiated by the contractions of the prostate, and it's a sensitive and erogenous gland. You can gently stimulate it by pressing the perineum, or more directly, by inserting a lubricated, clipped-nail finger up your anus, the procedure your doctor uses for a prostate exam (using a latex glove).

By finding the right spot on the perineum, described in Chia's *The Multi-Orgasmic Man* as the "million dollar spot,"[198] you can both stimulate your prostate and then inhibit ejaculation too.

Exercise

Specifically, your PC muscle. Here we arrive at Kegels again. See why we call them the king of all sexercise? Voluntarily contracting the PC muscles is another way to stop an ejaculation. Look in *Kegel* for specifics.

Breathe

Because breath rate increases as you approach your climax, slowing your breathing can help you move to and through orgasm without ejaculating. Breathing will also help you move the sexual energy away from the genitals and up the spine.

Meditate

Not the formal, cross-your-legs type, just the pay-attention-to-what's-happening awareness. Fantasy is fine, but this effort is about what's happening in your body, so switch back and be here for it. Try thinking about this sex as meditation, or if you prefer, this meditation as sex.

SPREAD THE AROUSAL

When you put all of the preceding together, you're ready to start experimenting with moving sexual energy up your spine to your brain and down the front of your body back to your genitals. The movement up concentrates and transforms the energy, making it available to your body and mind and not just your genitals; you can move it back down if and when the energy needs release. It's a healing process, and a pleasant one, as the sexual energy moves through the body.

Begin self-pleasuring, feeling the arousal in your genitals. Try inhaling, contracting your PC muscle, and anus, and imagine the sexual energy moving up your spine to your head. When making love with a woman and doing what you've practiced alone up to this point, you unite yin (feminine) and yang (masculine) energy, and both can experience enhanced pleasure and oneness.

TESTICLES

He's got balls.

Well, most men do. Yet it's a high-powered compliment—somehow the obvious anatomical fact has become high praise, testicles linked with serious courage and power and enhanced manliness.

Interesting. In fact, testicles are interesting for a variety of reasons. Granted, few people will swoon over their beauty. But take a few minutes to consider their importance, and you'll realize it's well worth the effort to spend a few moments a month examining them.

Any male who's taken a surprise knee or softball to the testicles knows about their sensitivity. That's Mother Nature's way of stressing their importance. After all, she's seriously concerned with reproduction.

You have to wonder why she designed sperm production for temperatures lower than the rest of your body. Whatever the reason, there they hang, exposed and up front. Maybe the courage association came about because men went forth and valiantly performed their appointed tasks despite this innate vulnerability.

Unfortunately most men don't give their testicles much attention in the absence of pain. Even though many won't suffer ill consequences as a result, some will. Hopefully after reading this chapter, you won't be among them. The simple truth is that you can vastly improve your chances of full recovery from a disease like testicular cancer by treating it early—and you'll know about it early when you learn and regularly practice a basic testicular self-exam. It's smart. It's simple. And we'll get to it right after sketching out the basic anatomy involved.

TESTICLES UP CLOSE AND PERSONAL

Is there a difference between testicles and testes and gonads? Yes. Gonads are sex organs that produce reproductive cells (both men and women have them). Testes (plural form of testis) are gonads of male vertebrates. Testicles are another name for testes, sometimes used to include the coiled tubes behind the testes, or simply the testes plus their scrotal sac.

Whatever you call them, their job remains the same. Testicles produce sperm and the male hormone testosterone. In a fetus they begin their journey near the abdomen and descend to their unique position in the eighth month of pregnancy. Occasionally they don't descend fully and surgeons intervene to make sure they do, because sperm production must take place down in the scrotum, due to temperature requirements. The scrotum is just a bit cooler than the rest of the body.

Roughly egg-shaped, with the feel of boiled eggs outside their shell, testicles come in all sizes and shapes, but average about two inches in length. According to Dr. Ken Goldberg, urologist and founder of the Male Health Center in Dallas, some men express concern regarding the size or shape of their testicles. Both naturally vary, he notes, but neither defines the state of your manliness![199]

The fact is, rather than dwelling on their appearance, men should be more concerned that their testicles stay healthy. Another doctor, Michael Oppenheim, author of *Man's Health Book*, notes that relative to women, men enjoy many years without needing anything corresponding to a regular gynecological exam.[200] That may account for the resistance many men feel about breaking down and going to a doctor's office to talk about a health concern. Getting a prescription for bronchitis or treating a pulled muscle is very different from asking someone to feel your left testicle.

And there's the rub. By the time doctors are asked about a health problem it can be advanced and much more dangerous than it would have been if reported earlier. As mentioned above, the first line of defense is a regular self-administered check. Here then are the basics for giving yourself a quick and easy Testicular Self-Examination, or TSE.

EXAMINE THEM REGULARLY

By the time a guy gets out of middle school he should be checking his testicles regularly. Why? Because testicular cancer, while a relatively rare disease, strikes mostly men aged 15 to 35. This is as good a time as any to get a sense of what's normal in an individual's body. Overall, the sooner a man adopts an active role in his own health care, the better health he's likely to enjoy later in life.

Get into the habit of a quick self-exam about once a month. Doing it on a particular day might help, maybe the first of the month, or whatever works for you. We're talking three minutes tops. So as an excuse, being too busy is pretty lame.

The best time to examine your testicles is during or after a shower or bath. The warmth relaxes your scrotum, making it easier to feel any abnormality. Try doing the exam while you're soaped up; you'll find that helps too.

Examine Your Testes

Start by taking one testicle between the thumb and first two fingers of each hand. Applying gentle pressure, roll the testicle between your fingers and check for lumps, which don't have to be painful to be noteworthy.

You may notice one testicle is larger than the other, or as you probably already know, one hangs lower than the other. Both of these are normal, although large differences in size should be noted.

Examine the Epididymis

Next, proceed to the epididymis, a coiled tube on the backside of each testicle. It stores sperm until it's ready to travel up the vas deferens to the urethra and out of the body. Generally more sensitive than the testis itself, the epididymis is also more likely to have a non-cancerous problem.

Examine the Vas Deferens

Again, the vas deferens is the tube leading from the testicles up to the staging area where ejaculation shoots sperm out of the body. In the scrotum, the tube should be smooth and firm.

What do you do if you have pain or notice anything out of the ordinary in the above steps? See your doctor. You may have any number of conditions, some less serious than others. Lumps, for instance, are generally not malignant. But since early treatment is definitely the keyword, there is absolutely no advantage here in being the strong silent type.

TESTICULAR PROBLEMS TO WATCH FOR

Since you've been doing your monthly exams, you have less to be concerned with regarding abnormalities. Nonetheless, here are the main categories of possible problems with the testicles that every man should know.

Testicular Cancer

Like other cancers, the testicular type is influenced by both genetic and environmental factors. Among the causes apparently not in play are sex or STD's.[201] One factor strongly correlated is undescended testicles, even in a testicle that descended normally when the other did not.

The most common symptom of testicular cancer is a lump, pain, or discomfort in the testicle, although other symptoms include aches in the groin or abdomen, or breasts that become enlarged or sensitive.

Whatever the cause, the primary goal is early detection, to treat as soon as possible and avoid the spread of cancer cells elsewhere in the body. Treatment will differ depending on whether it has spread. Type I stage tumors have remained in the testes; Type II have spread to lymph nodes close by; Type III have spread to more distant sites in the body. Diagnostic options range from ultrasound, X-rays, blood tests, biopsy, to surgical removal of the testes for examination. Treatment, depending on the type of cell affected, ranges from radiotherapy and chemotherapy, to surgery. Survival rates are good, especially for those cases involving early detection.

In addition to regular self-exams, ask your doctor about the advisability of a testicular exam in his regular physical examinations.

Benign Lumps or Swelling

Although some lumps or swellings in the testicles are not serious, you should obviously see your doctor to know for certain. Examples include:

- *hydrocele*

  A hydrocele is an accumulation of fluid which produces a swelling in the scrotum. It is painless and benign but should be examined nonetheless. A doctor may hold a light behind the scrotum to illuminate the clear fluid in the hydrocele and make sure there are no hidden tumors. No treatment is usually necessary.

- *Spermatocele*

  A spermatocele is a painless cyst filled with fluid, usually found above the testicle on the epididymis. Again not serious and usually left untreated.

- *Varicocele*

  Varicoceles are a thick varicose vein or veins found on the outside of a testicle. You may be more uncomfortable when standing because in lying down the pressure is relieved when blood drains. No treatment is necessary.

- *Hernia*

  Hernias affecting the scrotum result from a condition remaining from the time when testicles descended from the abdomen in the fetus. If the passage in which they descend remains open, part of the intestine can slip into the scrotum. This is the condition associated with "ball-busting" exertions. Although the condition can be remedied by simply pushing the intestine back where it belongs, it should be surgically repaired because complications can result from the intestine being caught and losing its blood supply.

Infections

- *Epididymitis*

    When a man registers pain in the testicle, an infection called epididymitis is most often the cause. Technically, the epididymis—not the testes—is the site of the infection. Often younger men get the offending bacteria through sexual contact; in older men a genitourinary tract infection is the more likely culprit. In both cases, antibiotics are prescribed.

- *Orchitis*

    When an infection does involve the testicle, the condition is called orchitis. It can arise from a bacterial infection, as described above in epididymitis, or a viral infection such as mumps. Most cases involve only one testicle. The bad news can be that after treatment (antibiotics) some testicles can shrink and lose fertility. The good news is that overall fertility is not affected by having only one testicle healthy.

Testicular Torsion

When pain in the testicles comes on suddenly, as opposed to the gradual onset of infection, torsion of the testicle is suspected. Basically, torsion results from the testicle being twisted, resulting in a crimp in the spermatic cord and its blood supply. The resulting pain can be intense, and the condition is serious because the testicle's blood supply is restricted. A doctor will try to simply untwist the testicle and cord, and if that fails surgery may be needed to reposition the testicle.

Testicular Trauma

When you land on the railing wrong, or get a bad hop and take a softball to the groin, you might sustain trauma, or injury, to a testicle. Fortunately the testes are tough resilient units, so that once the shock and pain wear off, you should be OK. But if an hour passes and you're still hurting, see a doctor. Prompt treatment can save a testicle that might otherwise develop complications.

THE JOY OF TESTICLES

Okay. Those are the conditions every man should know about. If you're fortunate you'll never have to deal with them. Now it's time to lighten up. Every man should tune into the sensuous nature of the family jewels, as some men affectionately refer to their testicles. When you and your lover are mapping a sex tour of each other's bodies, put your testicles on the itinerary. A definite erogenous zone, they're richly endowed with nerve endings connected to your brain's pleasure center.

In one survey of male sexuality, 67% of the sample reported testicles as the other part of their genital area that they like stimulated.[202]

Let your imagination be your guide, and encourage her to do the same. Testicles respond to being held, stroked, kissed, or otherwise appreciated and stimulated.

WHEN TO TUG YOUR TESTICLES

Although the technique is disputed by some, many men swear by using the testicles to delay orgasm. The theory is this: a man's testes elevate close to his body prior to ejaculation. By gently pulling the testicles down, ejaculation is inhibited and intercourse is prolonged. If your physical condition permits, your lover can try doing this, or when the intercourse position you're in allows it, you can try it yourself.

VARIETIES
OF SEXUAL EXPERIENCE

If sex was ordered from a menu, most Americans would choose meat and potatoes. Vaginal intercourse, and to a lesser degree oral sex, remain by far our central sexual acts.[203] But others enjoy different sexual fare, sampling more exotic dishes in restaurants off the beaten path.

Though morality seldom influences choices in food, it casts a long shadow over sex. Those who enjoy variants of the missionary position in heterosexual monogamy do so against the cultural grain.

Yet even the relatively conservative University of Chicago sex survey found that up to 9% of American men had at least one homosexual encounter since adolescence.[204] And up to 3% of men aged 18-44 find "being forced to do something sexual" appealing.[205]

While those percentages are relatively small, they translate into significant numbers of Americans who desire and/or practice offbeat varieties of sexual experience such as bondage, sadomasochism, and anal sex. Are they right or wrong? This book leaves moral judgments to others; the following survey of male sexuality explores what is, not what should be.

However, one of our basic sexual fitness guidelines does apply. If the practices described here do not generate mutual pleasure, they're out of bounds and a warning sign to both parties. This sex may be different, but like all good sex it must be consensual.

"SORRY, I'M TIED UP AND CAN'T COME TO THE PHONE RIGHT NOW..."

Every culture has defined roles for its members, which is a good thing; there would be chaos without them. The problem is, some roles are too narrowly defined for the whole person. A man's job, for example, might demand that he be constantly decisive and commanding. But that doesn't mean he might not like to show a more vulnerable side. There are many ways he might express that urge. Maybe sex in general is one; maybe bondage in particular is another, which could fit well with his partner if she wants to express more control in her life. Or vice versa.

Whatever the reasons, some people get excited by restraining and being restrained physically. They can get creative about it too — police handcuffs and a blindfold, special harnesses that fit around a bed or stick to the side of bathtubs, etc.

So what's it all about? Sometimes bondage is a mutual fantasy acted out to mutual pleasure. As noted in the *Fantasy* chapter, sexual imagination takes many forms, and making it real in role-playing can be a big turn-on. There's nothing wrong with you if you don't feel the urge to do so, nor if you do. But how safely you act it out is important.

Specifically, the thrill may flow from the dynamics of dominance and submission. Here's where the leather can emerge—along with parts of your personality banished by polite society. But whether the shared fantasy involves one costume or just two birthday suits, keep these ground rules in mind.

Keep it Comfortable

Start slowly. Try restraining your partner by command only, or by holding her arms or wrists in place. With her blindfolded, make suggestive suggestions. Tantalize. The fantasy should be a turn-on, not a turn-off—make sure she's into it. Then reverse roles and see how that feels.

Play it Safe

The goal is sexual excitement, not injury. Be careful that restraints aren't tied too tightly (learn alternatives to the common slip knot), or buy well-made cuffs, snaps, or clips from a sex boutique or mail order catalogs such as those listed in *Sex Toys*.

Agree on a word or sound that means an unequivocal stop in the action. Also, like driving, this is a time for sobriety. Don't leave anyone bound long enough for physical discomfort to set in. Trust must be at the heart of the play, because bondage usually involves a play of power, which we'll explore more specifically next.

WHO'S ON TOP?

S/M offers another excursion away from sexual boredom. Like the other sexual alternatives in this chapter, S/M can lead to enhanced arousal and orgasm simply because of the thrill of something new.

As in bondage, fantasy can play a major role. But the popular images of riding crops or spanking are not the whole picture. Though S/M is often associated with pain, in essence it's more about the dynamics of power.[206] Vulnerability, dominance, and submission can stir up powerful emotions which, when combined with sexual fantasies, can produce big time physical and psychological release.

At one extreme, the play becomes pain. Some people are attracted to the blurred boundary between pleasure and pain, and use elaborate leather outfits or special props like nipple clamps to get there. Again, and as long as it's absolutely consensual, that's a mutual decision wisely explored within the bounds of health concerns and common sense. After all, it's just one of many extreme human behaviors, like ironman training, which can move through various degrees of agony and gratification.

Other people are content to simply designate one partner as dominant and the other submissive, and explore the emotions and sexual sensations resulting from their respective roles. The only prop might be underwear to be ripped off. Or no props at all, just commands to be obeyed. If you're interested, watch a video to give you an idea of what intensity of S/M games, if any, appeals to you. Then find out if your sexual partner is interested, and then let your fantasies be your guide, or if you prefer, find a reliable guidebook such as *The New Good Vibrations Guide to Sex*, by Cathy Winks and Anne Semans.

Know in advance what sexual acts or props will be used. As in bondage, agree on safety rules like having a stop word or sound that won't be confused with the possibly illogical no's and yes's of passion.

TACTICAL REAR ACTIONS

Most people consider the anus to have only one function, which is elimination. But since it's an area richly endowed with nerve endings, which translate into pleasure, some sexual explorers find its pleasure a natural area to explore. One sex expert states that 30% of couples have given anal sex a go.[207]

The anus does not have a vagina's natural lubrication, so some form of lubrication must be used when penetrating or being penetrated. A condom is also a must when you are not absolutely sure that you and your partner are HIV-free (remember, the lube must be water-based for condom use).

As with other forms of sexual experience, anal sex offers a range of options, light to heavy, from gentle external stimulation to a vibrating sex toy on an internal mission. Some men over 40 have a surprise experience of anal pleasure during their first prostate exam. The doctor inserts his well-lubed finger and—hello!—the patient enjoys a feel-good sensation anally, sometimes accompanied by a stiff erection.

Depending on whether you already enjoy anal stimulation or find the very idea kinky beyond imagining, you may or may not be surprised to learn that a "vinyl butt plug is the number-one best-selling product of the nation's largest adult novelty manufacturer..."[208]

MEN AT PLAY

In our culture and others, many boys start their sexual life not with girls but with other boys. A very natural form of sex play, early same-gender sex avoids the complexity of between-gender relationships or fears of pregnancy, even though its easy playfulness is now complicated by the threat of AIDS among older participants.

Exactly how many men engage in homosexuality is difficult to say, starting with the difficulty of saying exactly what homosexuality is.[209] Some men have only one or two sexual encounters with other men. Others live for many years with one sexual orientation and change to another. Still others maintain sexual relationships with members of both sexes. And despite—or because of—the publicity in recent years involving gay men and the AIDS crisis, many men still keep their homosexuality private. Of course it would depend on where you consider, because in some cities the number would be quite large and in some rural areas, quite small.

There are many good books exploring male homosexuality in detail. While this book's focus is heterosexual sex, what follows is a brief look at what men do and don't do together and what it might mean for you.

STAY IN TOUCH

As we've seen elsewhere in this book, exactly what constitutes a sexual act, let alone sexual feelings, is not a black and white question. In a culture like ours, in which many men feel uncomfortable touching other men, the question is even more intense. Like the easy sexual play boys tend to engage in, men easily touching or embracing other men can become difficult for some men when adolescence passes.

But touching is a deeply satisfying act and in other cultures happens easily between men throughout life. Men walking arm in arm or kissing each other's cheeks are common. Sex therapist Bernie Zilbergeld, author of *The New Male Sexuality*, states that in our culture the simple comfort and support a man can naturally seek in touching other men can be the cause of inner conflict, and make him wonder if he has hidden homosexual tendencies.[210] The answer is found in a new, easier attitude. Be more accepting of your need for touch, counsels Zilbergeld, and satisfy it. Many feelings, including love, need not be linked with sex between men or women.

There is no definitive explanation of why some men are gay and some aren't. Some members of the scientific community seek to identify a "gay gene" while others focus on the imprint of personal experience in home and community. The gay liberation movement has helped many men come out and live comfortably with their sexuality. But sexual fantasies and desires for other men are not abnormal in heterosexual men, and they don't need to be acted out in the world. When those urges disrupt a man's life, however, it's time for him to talk to a trusted friend, family member or professional counselor to find out more about their meaning.

OUT OF THE ORDINARY

None of the above varieties of sexual experience are wrong, at least not in terms of two parties acting in mutual consent. But when any sexual desire or behavior causes difficulties at home, at work, or in the community, it crosses the line separating pleasurable and problematic. These problems may include the use of force, inappropriate behavior, or the necessity for certain scenarios or objects to enhance arousal and performance, including fetishism, exhibitionism, and rape. As fantasies, these are acceptable, but when they hurt a sexual relationship, or prevent an individual's ability to function without them, they are dangerous signposts of help needed, let alone actionable legal events.

Examples include *fetishism*, in which a sexualized object is necessary for arousal. Most men have enjoyed magazines featuring lingerie-clad women at one time or another. But when an object like feet or underwear need to be the center of attention for a man to get excited, then he's moved into the territory of paraphilias (literally "sex out of the ordinary") or the older label, perversion. Possibly in early sexual or emotional or physical abuse, sex was connected with something other than love and intimacy.

Voyeurism is the need to watch sex or sexual situations in order to be aroused. *Exhibitionism* requires exposing oneself to strangers and the risk of being caught. These and other addictive behaviors place a man outside the bounds of sexual fitness. They make sexual relationships difficult, and they can be difficult to change. For his sake and the sake of those with whom he's involved, a man struggling with these behaviors should seek professional counseling, which, like the aid of medical drugs, can help.

BIBLIOGRAPHY

Abdo, John, Dachman, Kenneth, *Body Engineering,* New York: The Berkley Publishing Group, 1997.

Abramson, Paul, Pinkerton, Steven, *With Pleasure,* New York: Oxford University Press, 1995.

American Council on Science and Health, *Cigarettes: What the Warning Label Doesn't Tell You,* New York, 1996.

Anand, Margo, *The Art of Sexual Ecstasy,* New York: Tarcher/Putnam, 1989.

Ashton, David, Davies, Bruce, *Why Exercise?,* New York: Basil Blackwell Inc., 1986.

Baldwin, Dorothy, *Understanding Male Sexual Health,* New York: Hippocrine Books, 1993.

Bechtel, Stephen, *The Practical Encyclopedia of Sex and Health,* Emmaus, PA: Rodale Press, 1993.

Belshin, Lee, *The Complete Prostate Book: Every Man's Guide,* Rocklin, CA: Prima Publishing, 1997.

Benson, Herbert, *The Relaxation Response,* New York: William Morrow and Company, 1975.

Berkowitz, Bob, *His Secret Life,* New York: Simon & Schuster, 1997.

Blue, Adrianne, *On Kissing,* New York: Kodansha International, 1997.

Blum, Deborah, *Sex on the Brain,* New York: Viking, 1997.

The Boston Women's Health Book Collective, *Our Bodies, Ourselves,* New York: Touchstone, 1998.

Bullough, Vern, Bullough, Bonne, *Sexual Attitudes,* Amherst, New York: Prometheus Books, 1995.

Castleman, Michael, *Sexual Solutions,* New York: Touchstone, 1989.

Chia, Mantak, Arava, Douglas, *The Multi-Orgasmic Man,* New York: HarperCollins, 1996.

Chia, Mantak, Winn, Michael, *Taoist Secrets of Love,* New York: Aurora Press, 1986.

Chopra, Deepak, *Healing the Heart,* New York: Harmony Books, 1998.

Cooper, Kenneth, *Dr. Kenneth Cooper's Antioxidant Revolution,* Nashville, TN: Thomas Nelson Inc., 1994.

Cooper, Robert, Cooper, Leslie, *Low-Fat Living,* Emmaus, PA: Rodale Press, Inc., 1996.

Crenshaw, Theresa, and Goldberg, James, *Sexual Pharmacology,* W.W. Norton & Company, New York, NY, 1996.

Dalai Lama, Cutler, Howard, *The Art of Happiness,* New York: Riverhead Books, 1998.

Danielou, Alain (translator), *The Complete Kama Sutra,* Rochester, VT: Park Street Press, 1994.

Diamond, Jed, *Male Menopause,* Naperville, IL: Sourcebooks, 1997.

Duke, James, *The Green Pharmacy,* Emmaus, PA: Rodale Press, 1997.

Feuerstein, Georg, *Tantra, The Path of Ecstasy,* Boston: Shambhala, 1998.

Garfinkel, Perry, Chichester, Brian, *Maximum Style: Look Sharp And Feel Confident In Every Situation,* Emmaus, PA: Rodale Press, 1997.

Giovannucci, Edward, et al, *The Journal of the American Medical Association,* February 17, 1993-vol. 269, No. 7.

Gittleman, Ann Louise, *Super Nutrition for Men,* New York: M. Evans and Company, Inc., 1996.

Goldberg, Ken, *How Men Can Live As Long As Women,* Fort Worth, Texas: The Summit Group, 1993.

Goleman, Daniel, *Emotional Intelligence,* New York: Bantam Books, 1995.

Goleman, Daniel, Gurin, Joel, editors, *Mind Body Medicine,* Yonkers, NY: Consumer Reports Books, 1993.

Greenberg, Jerrold, Bruess, Clint, Mullen, Kathleen, *Sexuality,* Dubuque, IA: Wm. D. Brown Communications, 1993.

Haas, Kurt, Haas, Adelaide, *Understanding Sexuality,* St. Louis: Mosby, 1993.

Hite, Shere, *The Hite Report on Male Sexuality,* New York: Alfred A. Knopf, 1981.

Hooper, Anne, *The Ultimate Sex Book,* London: Dorling Kindersley Limited, 1992.

Ivker, Robert, Zorensky, Edward, *Thriving,* New York: Crown Publishers, 1997.

Jung, C.G., *Aspects of the Masculine,* Princeton, NJ: Princeton University Press, 1989.

Jung, C.J., *Symbols of Transformation,* Princeton, NJ: Princeton University Press, 1956.

Keesling, Barbara, *Sexual Pleasure,* Alameda, CA: Hunter House, Inc., 1993.

Keville, Kathy, *Herbs for Health and Healing,* Emmaus, PA: Rodale Press, Inc., 1996.

Kinsey, Alfred, Pomeroy, Wardell, Martin, Clyde, *Sexual Behavior in the Human Male,* Philadelphia: W.B. Saunders Company, 1948.

Klitsch, Michael, *Vasectomy and Prostate Cancer: More Questions Than Answers,* Family Planning Perspectives, Vol. 25, No. 3, May/June 1993.

Kundtz, David, *Men and Feelings,* Deerfield Beach, FL: Health Communications, 1991.

Kybartas, Ray, *Fitness Is Religion,* New York: Simon and Schuster, 1997.

Lacroix, Nitya, Seager, Sharon, *The Book of Massage & Aromatherapy,* London: Lorenz Books, 1996.

Larson, David, *Mayo Clinic Family Health Book,* New York: William Morrow and Co.,1990.

Lazarus, Richard, Lazarus, Bernice, *Passion and Reason,* New York: Oxford University Press, 1994.

Leiblum, Sandra, Rosen, Raymond, *Sexual Desire Disorders,* New York: The Guilford Press, 1995.

Levant, Ronald, Kopecky, Gini, *Masculinity Reconstructed,* New York: Dutton, 1995.

Long, James, *The Essential Guide to Prescription Drugs,* New York: HarperCollins, 1993.

Margolies, Eva, *Undressing the American Male,* New York: Dutton, 1994

Mason, John, *Guide to Stress Reduction,* Berkeley, CA: Celestial Arts, 1985.

Masters, William, Johnson, Virginia, *Human Sexual Response,* New York: Bantam Books, 1966.

Michael, Robert, Gagnon, John, Laumann, Edward, and Kolata, Gina, *Sex In America,* Boston: Little, Brown and Co., 1994.

Moore, Thomas, *Soul Mates,* New York: HarperCollins, 1994.

Moore, Thomas, *The Soul of Sex,* New York: HarperCollins, 1998.

Morganstern, Steven, Abrahams, Allan, *Overcoming Impotence,* Englewood Cliffs, NJ: Prentice Hall, 1994.

Muir, Charles and Caroline, *Tantra, The Art of Conscious Living,* San Francisco: Mercury House, 1990.

Oppenheim, Michael, *The Man's Health Book,* Englewood Cliffs, NJ: Prentice Hall, 1994.

Puglio, Patricia, *"Male Menopause: Is It Real?",* *Life's Transitions,* Trumbull, CT: Broda Barnes, M.D. Research Foundation, Winter, 1997.

Reid, Daniel, *The Tao of Health, Sex, and Longevity,* New York: Fireside, 1989.

Reinisch, June, *The Kinsey Institute New Report on Sex,* New York: St. Martin's Press, 1990.

Rosen, Raymond, Leiblum, Sandra, *Case Studies in Sex Therapy,* New York: The Guilford Press, 1995.

Sahelian, Ray, *DHEA: A Practical Guide,* Garden City Park, NY: Avery Publishing Group, 1996.

Sanford, John, *Between People: Communicating One-to-One,* Mahwah, NJ: Paulist Press, 1988.

Schlosberg, Suzanne, Neporent, Liz, *Fitness For Dummies,* Foster City, CA: IDG Books Worldwide, 1996.

Schnarch, David, *Passionate Couples,* New York: W. W. Norton & Co., 1997.

Sears, Barry, *The Zone,* New York: Harper Collins, 1995.

Sheehy, Gail, *Understanding Men's Passages,* New York: Random House, 1998.

USPDI, *Drug Information For The Health Care Professional,* Rockville, MD: United States Pharmacopial Convention, 1995.

Walker, Lynne, Brown, Ellen, *Nature's Pharmacy,* Paramus, NJ: Prentice Hall, 1998.

Walker, Morton, *Sexual Nutrition,* Garden City Park, NY: Avery Publishing Group, 1994.

Weil, Andrew, *Eight Weeks to Optimum Health,* New York: Alfred A. Knopf, Inc., 1997.

Welwood, John, *Challenge of the Heart,* Boston: Shambhala, 1985.

Winks, Cathy, Semans, Anne, *The New Good Vibrations Guide To Sex,* San Francisco: Cleis Press Inc., 1997.

Winter, Ruth, *A Consumer's Dictionary of Medicines,* New York: Crown Publishers, 1993.

Yaffé, Maurice, Fenwick, Elizabeth, *Sexual Happiness for Men,* New York: Henry Holt and Company, 1992.

Yeager, Selene, *New Foods for Healing,* Emmaus: PA, Rodale Press, Inc, 1998.

Zilbergeld, Bernie, *The New Male Sexuality,* Bantam Books, New York, NY, 1992.

NOTES

[1] James McCary and Stephen McCary, *Human Sexuality* (Belmont, CA: Wadsworth, 1982), page 56.

[2] Tamar Nordenberg, "From Anchovies to Oysters: Do Aphrodisiacs Really Work?," *FDA Consumer*, Jan-Feb, 1996.

[3] James Duke, *The Green Pharmacy* (Emmaus, PA: Rodale Press, 1997), p. 189.

[4] Ibid, p. 188.

[5] Adapted from Kurt Haas and Adelaide Haas, *Understanding Sexuality* (St. Louis: Mosby, 1993), p. 353.

[6] SIECUS, "The Truth about Latex Condoms," New York, *FACTSHEET* 1997.

[7] Path, *Outlook*, "Emergency Contraceptive Pills: Safe and Effective But Not Widely Used," September, 1996, http://www.path.org/html/14_2_fea.htm.

[8] Ibid, SIECUS.

[9] Edward Giovannucci, et al, "A Prospective Cohort Study of Vasectomy and Prostate Cancer," *The Journal of the American Medical Association,* February 17, 1993—vol. 269, No. 7, page 873.

[10] Michael Klitsch, "Vasectomy and Prostate Cancer: More Questions Than Answers," *Family Planning Perspectives*, Volume 25, No. 3 May/June 1993, page 134.

[11] Society for the Advancement of Education, *USA Today* (Magazine), February 1995, p. 12.

[12] Steve Sternberg, "Reproductive Equality: A Male Pill?," *Science News,* 6/22/96, p. 388.

[13] Bernie Zilbergeld, *The New Male Sexuality* (New York: Bantam Books, 1993), p. 330.

[14] Anne Hooper, *The Ultimate Sex Book* (London: Dorling Kindersley Limited, 1992), p. 101.

[15] Robert Michael, John Gagnon, Edward Laumann, Gina Lolata, *Sex in America,* New York: Little Brown, 1994, p. 25.

[16] Zilbergeld, p. 340.

17 Walker, p. 137.

18 Zilbergeld, p. 443.

19 Michael Oppenheim, *The Man's Health Book* (Englewood Cliffs, NJ: Prentice Hall, 1994), p. 256.

20 Ibid, p. 256.

21 Mantak Chia, Douglas Arava, *The Multi-Orgasmic Man* (San Francisco: HarperCollins, 1996, p. 46.

22 Maurice Yaffé, Elizabeth Fenwick, *Sexual Happiness For Men* (New York: Henry Holt and Company, 1992), p. 90.

23 Michael Castleman, *Sexual Solutions* (New York: Touchstone, 1989), p. 86.

24 David Schnarch, *Passionate Couples* (New York: W.W. Norton, 1997), p. 160.

25 Daniel Goleman, *Emotional Intelligence* (New York: Bantam Books, 1995), p. 6.

26 Adapted from David Kundtz, *Men and Feelings* (Deerfield Beach, FL: Health Communications, Inc., 1991), p. 88.

27 Ronald Levant, *Masculinity Reconstructed* (New York: Dutton, 1995), p. 230.

28 Goleman, p. 171.

29 Ibid, p. 177.

30 Richard Lazarus, Bernice Lazarus, *Passion and Reason* (New York: Oxford University Press, 1994), p. 20.

31 Walker, p. 135.

32 Alex Markels, "Woe is Us," *Men's Journal,* October 1998, p. 137.

33 Walker, p. 136.

34 Selene Yeager, *New Foods for Healing* (Emmaus: PA, Rodale Press, 1998), p. 178.

35 Alan Cohen, Barbara Bartlik, "Ginkgo Biloba for Antidepressant-Induced Sexual Dysfunction," *Journal of Sex & Marital Therapy,* 24:139-143, p. 139.

36 Maurice Yaffé, Elizabeth Fenwick, *Sexual Happiness for Men* (New York: Henry Holt and Company, 1992), p. 69.

37 Levant, p. 85.

38 The Dalai Lama and Howard Cutler, *The Art of Happiness,* New York: Riverhead Books, 1998, p. 13.

39 Lazarus, p. 90.

40 Ray Kybartas, *Fitness Is Religion,* New York: Simon and Schuster, 1997, p. 117.

41 David Ashton and Bruce Davies, *Why Exercise?* (New York: Basil Blackwell Inc, 1986), p. 94.

42 *Sexual Fitness* (Alexandria, VA: Time Life Books, 1988), p. 9.

43 Ibid, p. 16.

44 Robert Goldman, "Exercise: The Ultimate Anti-aging pill," *TotalHealth for Longevity,* Vol. 20, Num. 3, p. 11.

45 Dr. Ken Goldberg, *How Men Can Live As Long As Women* (Fort Worth, Texas: The Summit Group, 1993), p. 97.

46 Dr. Kenneth Cooper, *Dr. Kenneth Cooper's Antioxidant Revolution* (Nashville, TN: Thomas Nelson Inc., 1994), p. 57.

47 Kybartas, p. 180.

48 Abdo and Dachman, p. 21.

49 Bob Berkowitz, *His Secret Life* (New York: Simon & Schuster, 1997), p. 15.

50 Carl Jung, *Symbols of Transformation,* Princeton, NJ: Princeton University Press, 1956, p. 29.

51 Ibid, p. 310.

52 "Eroticism and Gender," *U.S. News & World Report,* 7/19/93, p. 62-3.

53 June Reinisch, *The Kinsey Institute New Report on Sex* (New York: St. Martin's Press, 1990), p. 93.

54 Nancy Friday, *My Secret Garden* (New York: Simon & Schuster, 1973), p. 3.

55 Yaffé, p. 121.

56 Joseph Pissorno, *Total Wellness* (Rocklin, CA: Prima Publishing, 1996), p. 257.

57 Haas and Haas, p. 74-75, 100-107, 242-3.

58 http://www.resolve.org/started/htm

59 Reinisch, p. 312.

[60] Ibid, p. 310.

[61] http://www.resolve.org/started/htm

[62] Egbert Velde, Bernard Cohlen, "The Management of Infertility," *New England Journal of Medicine,* 1/21/99, Vol. 340, No. 3.

[63] Shere Hite, *The Hite Report on Male Sexuality* (New York: Alfred A. Knopf, 1981), p. 1113-4.

[64] http://www.sexuality.org/aspp.html

[65] www. sugarplums.com/ezine/research4.html (reporting research from the Smell and Taste Research and Treatment Foundation).

[66] Michael Oppenheim, *The Man's Health Book* (Englewood Cliffs, NJ: Prentice Hall, 1994), p. 183.

[67] http://www.swmed.edu/ home_pages/library/ consumer/ dryskin.htm

[68] Neil D. Rosenberg, *Milwaukee Journal Sentinel,* "Cologne Can Turn A Head—Or A Stomach," *Denver Rocky Mountain News,* 8/3/98, p. 4D.

[69] http:// www. learn2.com/05/0566

[70] http://www.aad.org/P_Frameset.htmlHAIRLOSS

[71] Deborah Blum, *Sex on the Brain* (New York: Viking, 1997), p. 168.

[72] Ken Flieger, *"Testosterone: Key to Masculinity and More,"* FDA Consumer (May 1995, volume 29), p. 29.

[73] Mayo Clinic, "Testosterone Replacement," Mayo Health Oasis, 8/16/96.

[74] Ronald Klatz and Robert Goldman, *"When a Man's Sex Drive Wanes: Is Testosterone the Answer?"* Sexual Health, Issue #1, p. 39.

[75] *"Low Testosterone Levels Can Alter Prostate Tests,"* Minneapolis Star Tribune, 2/2/97, p. 3E.

[76] Ibid, p. 38.

[77] Ray Sahelian, *DHEA, A Practical Guide* (Garden City Park, NY: Avery Publishing Group, 1996), page 5.

[78] Therese Crenshaw, James Goldberg, *Sexual Pharmacology* (New York: W.W. Norton Co., 1996), p. 43.

[79] *"Testosterone shots fight effects of age, but won't recapture youth, doctor says,"* Minneapolis Star Tribune, 11/7/96, Page 3E.

[80] Goldberg, p. 53.

[81] Gail Sheehy, *"Understanding Men's Passages* (New York: Random House, 1998), p. 195.

[82] J.B. Saunders, *"Alcohol: an important cause of hypertension,"* British Medical Journal, 1987, 294, p. 1045-6.

[83] Nicholas Emanuele and Mary Ann Emanuele, *"The endocrine system: alchohol alters critical hormonal balance..."* Alcohol Health & Research World, Vol. 21, 1997, p. 53.

[84] The American Council on Science and Health, *Cigarettes, What the Warning Label Doesn't Tell You* (New York, 1996), p. 98.

[85] "Pfizer Updates Viagra Labeling," (FDA Talk Paper, Rockville, MD) 11/4/98.

[86] Hite, p. 1102.

[87] David Schnarch, *Passionate Couples* (New York: W. W. Norton & Co., 1997), p. 261.

[88] John Gray, *Mars and Venus in the Bedroom* (New York: HarperCollins, 1997), p. 77.

[89] Reinisch, p. 118.

[90] The Boston Women's Health Book Collective, *Our Bodies, Ourselves* (New York: Touchstone, 1998), p. 256.

[91] "Want a Healthier Heart? Make Love More Often; Dr. Dean Ornish Also Endorses Intimacy," *Business Wire*, 10/7/98.

[92] David Schnarch, *Passionate Couples* (New York: W. W. Norton & Co., 1997) p. 101.

[93] John Welwood, *Challenge of the Heart* (Boston: Shambhala, 1985), p. 18.

[94] Thomas Moore, *Soul Mates* (New York: HarperCollins,1994), p. 24.

[95] Schnarch, p. 38.

[96] Dalai Lama, Howard Cutler, *The Art of Happiness*, pp. 78-9.

[97] Schnarch, p. 153.

[98] John Welwood, *Challenge of the Heart* (Boston: Shambhala Publications, 1985), p. 66.

[99] Adrianne Blue, *On Kissing,* (New York: Kodansha International).

[100] Alain Danielou (translator), *The Complete Kama Sutra* (Rochester, VT: Park Street Press, 1994), p. 126.

[101] Elliot Greene, *"Massage Therapy for Health and Fitness,"* http://www. doubleclickd.com/theramassage.html

[102] Nitya Lacroix, *Sensual Massage* (New York: Henry Holt and Company, 1989), p. 9.

[103] Robert T. Michael, John H. Gagnon, Edward O. Laumann, and Gina Kolata, *Sex in America, A Definitive Survey* (Little, Brown and Company, 1994), p. 165.

[104] Hoag Levins, *American Sex Machines: The Hidden History of Sex at the U.S. Patent Office*.

[105] Brown Walker, p. 4.

[106] C.G Jung, *Aspects of the Masculine* (Princeton, NJ: Princeton University Press, 1989), p. 25.

[107] Jed Diamond, *Male Menopause* (Napierville, IL: Sourcebooks, 1997), p. 90.

[108] The American Council on Science and Health, *Cigarettes, What the Warning Label Doesn't Tell You* (New York, 1996), p. 96.

[109] Bernie Zilbergeld, *The New Male Sexuality* (New York: Bantam Books, 1992), p. 585.

[110] Walker, p. 136.

[111] Gail Sheehy, *Understanding Men's Passages* (New York: Random House, 1998), p. 195.

[112] C.G. Jung, p. 29.

[113] Shere Hite, *The Hite Report on Male Sexuality* (New York: Ballantine Books, 1987) p. 866.

[114] Daniel Goleman and Joel Gurin, editors, *Mind Body Medicine* (Yonkers, NY: Consumer Reports Books, 1993), p. 23.

[115] Deborah Blum, *Sex on the Brain* (New York: Viking, 1997).

[116] Barry McCarthy, "Strategies and Techniques for Revitalizing a Nonsexual Marriage," *Journal of Sex & Marital Therapy,* Vol. 23, no. 3, p. 231.

[117] David Schnarch, *Passionate Couples* (New York: W.W. Norton & Co., 1997) p. 76.

[118] Schnarch, p. 80.

[119] Morton Walker, *Sexual Nutrition* (Garden City Park, NY: Avery Publishing Group, 1994), p. 27.

[120] K. Khaw, E. Barrett-Conner, "Dietary Potassium and Stroke-Associated Mortality," New England Journal of Medicine 316(5): 235-40, 1987.

[121] Ming Wei, et al. "Total Cholesterol and High Density Lipoprotein Cholesterol as Important Predictors of Erectile Dysfunction." *American Journal of Epidemiology*. 1994; 140: 930-7.

[122] Walker, ibid, p. 51.

[123] Ann Louise Gittleman, *Super Nutrition for Men* (New York: M. Evans and Company, Inc., 1996), p. 65.

[124] Robert Cooper, Leslie Cooper, *Low Fat Living* (Emmaus, PA: Rodale Press), 1996.

[125] Ibid, p. 12.

[126] Lynne Walker, p. 218.

[127] Lynne Walker, p. 282.

[128] Andrew Weil, *Eight Weeks to Optimum Health* (New York: Alfred A. Knopf, 1997), p. 49.

[129] Meir Stampfer, M. Malinow, "Can Lowering Homocysteine Levels Reduce Cardiovascular Risk?," *The New England Journal of Medicine,* Volume 332, #5, 2/2/95.

[130] David Larson, M.D., *Mayo Clinic Family Health Book* (New York: William Morrow and Co., 1990), p. 368.

[131] Andrew Weil, *Eight Weeks to Optimum Health* (New York: Alfred A. Knopf, Inc., 1997), p. 85.

[132] Kathy Keville, *Herbs for Health and Healing* (Emmaus, PA: Rodale Press, Inc., 1996), p. 195.

[133] Morton Walker, p. 52.

[134] James Duke, *The Green Pharmacy* (Emmaus, PA: Rodale Press, 1997), p. 188.

[135] *The American Journal of Natural Medicine*, Vol. 1, No. 1, September 1994.

[136] Stephanie A. Sanders, June Machover Reinisch, "Would You Say You 'Had Sex' If...," JAMA, 1/20/99, Vol. 281, No. 3, p. 275.

[137] Cathy Winks, Anne Semans, *The New Good Vibrations Guide to Sex* (San Francisco: Cleis Press, Inc., 1997), p. 84.

[138] Michael, et al, *Sex in America*, p. 146.

[139] Reinisch, p. 132.

[140] http://www.sexuality.org/l/incoming/ghoas.html (this is the excellent sexuality.org site at the University of Washington).

[141] Jerrold Greenberg, Clint Bruess, Kathleen Mullen, *Sexuality* (Dubuque, IA: Wm. D. Brown Communications, 1993), p. 623.

[142] Hite, p. 1117.

[143] Mantak Chia, Douglas Abrams Arava, *The Multi-Orgasmic Man* (New York: HarperCollins, 1996), p. 26.

[144] Stephen Bechtel, *The Practical Encyclopedia of Sex and Health* (Emmaus, PA: Rodale Press, 1993), p. 257.

[145] Goldberg, p. 181.

[146] Paul Abramson, Steven Pinkerton, *With Pleasure* (New York: Oxford University Press, 1995), p. 199.

[147] Vern Bullough, Bonne Bullough, *Sexual Attitudes* (Amherst, New York: Prometheus Books, 1995), p. 190.

[148] Castleman, p. 195.

[149] Lee Belshin, *The Complete Prostate Book* (Rocklin, CA: Prima Publishing, 1997). p. 9.

[150] "Prostate Cancer and Green Tea," 1/12/99, http://www.mayohealth.org/mayo/9901/htm/tea.htm

[151] Henry Miller, *The World of Sex* (New York: Grove Press, 1978), p. 107.

[152] Jill Neimark, "The Beefcaking of America" (*Psychology Today*, Vol. 27, 11/1/94), p. 32.

[153] Alfred Kinsey, Wardell Pomeroy, Clyde Martin, *Sexual Behavior in the Human Male* (Philadelphia: W.B. Saunders Company, 1948), p. 158.

[154] Ibid, p. 164.

[155] Ibid, p. 195.

[156] Ibid, p. 238.

[157] William Masters, Virginia Johnson, *Human Sexual Response* (New York: Bantam Books), 1966.

[158] Ibid, p. 4.

[159] Ibid, p. 192.

[160] Shere Hite, *The Hite Report of Male Sexuality* (New York: Random House, 1978), p. 1098.

[161] Robert Michael et al, *Sex in America.*

[162] Ibid, p. 92.

[163] Ibid, p. 246.

[164] Eva Margolies, *Undressing the American Male* (New York: Dutton, 1994), p. 20.

[165] Raymond Rosen, Sandra Leiblum, *Case Studies in Sex Therapy* (New York: The Guilford Press, 1995), p. 23.

[166] Margolies, p. 179.

[167] Ibid, p. 65.

[168] Ibid, p. 75.

[169] Margolies, p. 27.

[170] Michael et al, *Sex In America*, p. 147.

[171] "Toys in the Sheets," http://www.xandria.com.

[172] Winks and Semans, p. 96.

[173] Margo Anand, *The Art of Sexual Ecstasy* (New York: Tarcher/Putnam, 1989), p. 201.

[174] David Schnarch, "Joy with Your Underwear Down," *Psychology Today*, Vol. 27, 7/1/94, p. 39.

[175] Michael et al, *Sex in America,* p. 116.

[176] Ibid, p. 113.

[177] Chia, p. 79.

[178] Oren J. Cohen, Anthony S. Fauci, "HIV/AIDS in 1998—Gaining the Upper Hand?", *Journal of the American Medical Association*, July 1, 1998.

[179] http://aepo-xdv-www.epo.cdc.gov//wonder/prevguid

[180] L. John Mason, *Guide to Stress Reduction* (Berkeley, CA: Celestial Arts: 1985), p. 4.

[181] Ibid, p. 3.

[182] Sheehy, p. 87.

[183] Herbert Benson, *The Relaxation Response,* New York: William Morrow and Company, 1975.

[184] Lynne Walker, p. 136.

[185] Keville, p. 55.

[186] Goleman and Gurin, p. 31.

[187] Ibid, p. 29.

[188] Margo Anand, p. 47.

[189] Georg Feuerstein, *Tantra, the Path of Ecstasy* (Boston: Shambhala, 1998), p. 228.

[190] Charles and Caroline Muir, *Tantra, The Art of Conscious Living* (San Francisco: Mercury House), p. 17.

[191] Anand, p. 163.

[192] Feuerstein, p. 32.

[193] Alan Watts, *Tao, The Watercourse Way* (New York: Pantheon), 1975, p. 41.

[194] Ibid, p. 87.

[195] Mantak Chia and Michael Winn, *Taoist Secrets of Love* (New York: Aurora Press, 1986), p. 32.

[196] Daniel Reid, *The Tao of Health, Sex, and Longevity* (New York: Fireside, 1989), p. 288.

[197] Mantak Chia, Douglas Abrams Arava, *The Multi-Orgasmic Man* (New York: HarperCollins, 1996), p. 17-18.

[198] Ibid, p. 51.

[199] Goldberg, p. 148.

[200] Oppenheim, p. 151.

[201] Ibid, p. 152.

[202] Hite, p. 1111.

[203] Michael et al, *Sex In America*, p. 146.

[204] Ibid, p. 175.

[205] Ibid, p. 147.

[206] Winks and Semans, p. 210.

[207] Zilbergeld, p. 123.

[208] Winks and Semans, p. 162.

[209] Michael et al, p. 172.

[210] Zilbergeld, p. 304.

INDEX

A

Abstinence, 26
Acne, 91
Adrenaline, 97
Aerobic training, 58-61
Afterglow, 1, 3-4
Aftershock, 2
AIDS, 241-242
Alcohol, 150
    abuse, medication for, 145
    and ED, 102
Alexithymia, 44
Alternative medications, 150-151
American Sex Machines, 139
Anal sex, 271-272
Anger, 48-50
    controlling, 49
    during midlife, 155
Anonymous sex, 72-73
Anti-aging, 98-99
    and Taoism, 260
Antidepressants, 5, 30, 51
Anxiety, 32, 50, 52
    medications for, 145
Aphrodisiacs, 5-10, 34
Aromatherapy, 134
Arousal, 83-84
    by kissing, 130
    stages of, 1, 220
Artificial insemination, 82
Attitudes
    and lack of desire, 34
    of losers/winners, 15

B

Bathing together, 4
Benign Prostatic Hyperplasia (BPH), 199
Berkowitz, Bob, 71
Birth control pill, male, 27-28
Birth control

and oral sex, 177
male pill, 27-28
See also Contraceptives
Blood pressure medicine, 30
Bondage, 233, 269-270
Breath, preventing halitosis, 94-95

C

Cancer,
    testicular, 265-266
    medications for, 145
    prostate, 200
Carbohydrates, 167
Cardiovascular disease
    and diet, 166-167
    and viagra, 143
    medications for, 146
Chakras, 256
Champagne, 6
Chancroid, 244
Chia, Mantak, 39, 186, 259
Chlamydia, 242-243
Chocolate, 6
Cholesterol, 169-170
Cleanliness, 95
Clitoris, 183
Coitus interruptus, 25
Coitus, *See* Intercourse
Cologne, male, 91
Communication, 16-21
    after sex, 2-3
    by touch, 132-133
    game, 17
    in monogamous relationship, 157
    silent, 19-21
    tips, 17-18
Condoms, 23-25
Confidence, and sex appeal, 212
Consent, between partners, 12, 273-274
Contraceptives, 23-28
    and lack of desire, 35
Cooper, Dr. Kenneth, 63